SURVIVAL GUIDE

for the
BEGINNING
SPEECH-LANGUAGE
CLINICIAN

Susan Moon Meyer, PhD
Department of Special Education
Division of Speech-Language Pathology
Kutztown University
Kutztown, Pennsylvania

AN ASPEN PUBLICATION®
Aspen Publishers, Inc.
Gaithersburg, Maryland
1998

Library of Congress Cataloging-in-Publication Data

Meyer, Susan Moon.
Survival guide for the beginning speech-language clinician/ Susan
Moon Meyer.
p. cm.
Includes bibliographical references and index.
ISBN 0-8342-1116-5
1. Speech therapy—Practice. 2. Speech therapy. I Title.
[DNLM: 1. Language Disorders—therapy. 2. Speech Disorders—therapy.
3. Speech-Language Pathology—methods. WL 340.2M613s
1998]
RC428.5.M49   1998
616 85´506—dc21
DNLM/DLC
for Library of Congress
98-27314
CIP

Aspen Publishers, Inc., grants permission for photocopying for limited personal or internal use.
This consent does not extend to other kinds of copying, such as copying for general distribution, for
advertising or promotional purposes, for creating new collective works, or for resale. For information, address Aspen Publishers, Inc., Permissions Department, 200 Orchard Ridge Drive, Suite 200,
Gaithersburg, Maryland 20878.

Orders: (800) 638-8437
Customer Service: (800) 234-1660

About Aspen Publishers • For more than 35 years, Aspen has been a leading professional
publisher in a variety of disciplines. Aspen's vast information resources are available in both
print and electronic formats. We are committed to providing the highest quality information
available in the most appropriate format for our customers. Visit Aspen's Internet site for more
information resources, directories, articles, and a searchable version of Aspen's full catalog,
including the most recent publications: **http://www.aspenpublishers.com**
Aspen Publishers, Inc. • The hallmark of quality in publishing
Member of the worldwide Wolters Kluwer group.

Editorial Services: Kathleen Ruby
Library of Congress Catalog Card Number: 98-27314
ISBN: 0-8342-1116-5

Printed in the United States of America

TO THE STUDENT

Nothing is as moving as the expression of gratitude expressed by a newly discharged child's gift of flowers to the clinician, as shown on the back cover. It symbolizes not the end of the process but, for the client, the beginning of a new life. This is the best reason to endure your arduous education and clinical training—the opportunity to bring joy and wonder to those who may have believed that their lives would hold neither.

To my husband for his unending love, guidance, suggestions, and support
To our children for their continuing love and challenge
To my students for their inspiration

Table of Contents

Preface

The *Survival Guide for the Beginning Speech-Language Clinician* is intended as a supplemental text for when you take your first steps toward a career as a speech-language pathologist. Regardless of whether you are an undergraduate or graduate student, this book is useful to everyone undertaking their first clinical experience. The goals of this book are to provide you with a realistic, practical, and comprehensive overview of clinical problems that are often encountered by beginning clinicians and then to present solutions to those problems. This book does not focus on the numerous principles and theories that underlie various aspects of the clinical process because these are covered for you in the classroom.

Although the intent just stated is the primary purpose of this book, a secondary purpose has surfaced during the writing of this manuscript. This book can also assist the newest segment of our profession—speech-language pathology assistants—as they journey through their training programs. Although speech-language pathology assistants differ from speech-language clinicians in terms of educational requirements and scope of responsibilities, they will still have to complete practicum under the supervision of an American Speech-Language-Hearing Association (ASHA)-certified speech-language pathologist. Having pointed this out, what follows is a discussion of what you will find in this book.

The Introduction includes the rationale for writing this book. My former students' comments regarding feelings, attitudes, and perceptions toward the clinical practicum procedure are included to help you realize that your apprehensions are not unique. Three groups of students performing at different levels of the clinical process are identified, and the major clinical problem encountered by each group is addressed to show you how you will progress and what will be expected of you.

The importance of writing behavioral objectives is stressed in chapter 1. The three components of a behavioral objective are discussed, and examples pertinent to each component are presented. Relevant examples of various communication problems encountered in the profession of speech-language pathology are given.

Opportunities will be provided for you to identify the performance, condition, and criterion portions of objectives. The importance of understanding and writing behavioral objectives is discussed.

Chapter 2 is based on this author's more than 20 years of experience in reading, correcting, revising, rewriting, and approving behavioral objectives that were written by many hundreds of former beginning clinicians. Frequent problems in designing behavioral objectives are provided and discussed in an attempt to prevent you from repeating the same mistakes.

The purpose of chapter 3 is to make you aware of the necessity of writing well-written evaluations. This is achieved by first presenting and analyzing an evaluation that is poorly written. General guidelines are provided for writing both professional-style evaluations and progress reports. Organization as well as content is emphasized.

Chapter 4 contains samples of evaluations, re-evaluations, and progress reports that are well written. It is possible for you to experience the flow and style of professional writing by actively reading and rereading these samples. Additional guidelines for writing professional reports are provided.

Writing progress notes in a professional manner is the focus of chapter 5. Information and examples designed to stimulate your thinking and analytical skills are provided to help you write acceptable progress notes. Examples of both acceptable and problematic progress note entries are presented and discussed. Suggestions for improvement are provided when necessary. You will discover that progress notes are not ends in themselves but should be scrutinized and used to help determine the flow and direction of the therapeutic program.

Chapter 6 addresses several aspects of clinical accountability that are important to beginning clinicians. The first aspect involves the paperwork process. An efficient system for handling the voluminous amount of paperwork expected of you is described, and a rationale is presented. Record-keeping during therapy sessions is also a focus. Examples, problems, suggestions, and samples of record-keeping systems are presented and discussed. An emphasis is also placed on keeping track of clinical hours. The types of activities that should be recorded in clinical hours is discussed and presented in a check-sheet format.

The purpose of chapter 7 is to offer suggestions to make your therapeutic sessions run more smoothly and to enable you to perform more efficiently and effectively during the clinical process. The content of this chapter is based on frequently occurring problematic areas noted during observations of former beginning clinicians. By identifying problems, showing how they can interfere with the effectiveness of the therapeutic process, and providing solutions, it is hoped that you will avoid these common pitfalls. Helpful hints to enhance performance are presented and discussed. Some areas that are discussed are seating arrangement, reinforcement for therapy and testing, verbal models, smothering the client, fostering dependency, choice constancy, reading sequence, elicitation techniques, use of questions sparingly, avoidance of being physically overpowering, directions, receptive tasks, group therapy, elimination of habits that may be misinterpreted, avoidance of game emphasis, carryover, sign language, session opening, and session closing.

The eighth chapter encourages you to evaluate consciously and continuously all aspects of your professional performance. Some simple techniques are presented to help you begin to evaluate your own clinical performance. Basic clinical behaviors, which need to be addressed when evaluating your sessions, are presented and discussed. Additionally, abstract and complex clinical behaviors are presented, as you need to incorporate them into your self-evaluations. These are also the behaviors that will be evaluated by most of your supervisors.

It is important to underscore a few points. The names and addresses of clients and agencies have been changed to protect their identity. The actual year in which various clinical events occurred is not given in order to prevent this book from immediately becoming obsolete. Although "beginning" does not always precede "clinician," the intent is that nearly all references to "clinician" in this book are to the beginning clinician. When this is not true, the meaning should be obvious from the context. Initially an attempt was made to refer to clinicians as "he" or "she" or "him" or "her" as appropriate. However socially correct, this is frequently dropped in favor of referring to clinicians as female and clients (most often) as male because it made the text less awkward and because this better reflects the statistical reality of the profession. I trust this will not offend you.

Another convention adopted here is to enclose sample documents (or portions thereof) within a border. Although this does not fully "simulate" the document, it will serve to alert you to whether you are still reading within a document or have returned to the text. ("Quick Checks" and reviews are also boxed, but they will be obvious to you as you use them. Please do use them, as they can alert you to topics you may need to review more thoroughly.) Also understand that presentation of headings and subheadings may differ within the sample documents compared with the format used in this book. This should not be seen as a fault but a by-product of moving between two methods in the acquisition of knowledge: theory and practice. Both sources of information are needed in any educational endeavor.

In the area of knowledge acquisition and application, the profession of speech-language pathology continues to benefit from the continuing evolution of information-based technology. Augmentative devices and computer software are readily available to assist with all aspects of the clinical process (administration, diagnosis, treatment, report writing, and so forth). It is not the intent to ignore the great impact of this technology; however, you will be better able to select and utilize available technology, and to understand and appreciate better the value of computers and software, if you first experience the clinical process without the aid of this technology. Experiencing the clinical process in this manner will enable you to understand it better, to evaluate your needs, and ultimately, to be more knowledgeable of the technology you may require. For these reasons, the use of computer technology is not further addressed in this book. In a sense, being a good clinician rests on your shoulders and not in a keyboard or mouse.

This author's understanding of how you can be successful in speech-language pathology continues to grow. It is the author's intent that this book will stimulate everyone (supervisors, former beginning clinicians, and so on) using it to explore additional ways to help future beginning clinicians have an easier more enjoyable initial experience—an experience that not only ends, but also begins, with them delighting in their new clinical roles.

There are many people to whom thanks are owed. Sincere thanks go to all the students whom I have supervised. Thank you for all I have learned from you. To John C. Meyer, Jr., my husband, thank you for the great photographs! To Ellen Kwiatkowski, thank you for information and support! To Rusty (Ronald) Miller, thank you for designing the cartoons. Appreciation is expressed to the following clinical supervisors who took the time to read and comment on the first draft: Ellen Cohn, Rich Forcucci, Peggy Goll, Kathy Linnan, Bob Lowe, Frank McPherson, Loline Saras, Esther Shane, Elaine Shuey, Elena Stuart, and Kelly Webb. Thanks are also due to the external reviewers for, and the fine professionals of, Aspen Publishers. Their comments resulted in a better draft. Above all, a very special thank you goes to my husband John and to our children, Chris and Scott, who were very supportive and endured my preoccupation with this book. John's numerous readings of this material and gentle suggestions were greatly appreciated!

Introduction: A Discussion on "Bridging the Gap"—Taking Your First Step toward Obtaining Professional Status

DIFFERENT NEEDS FOR DIFFERENT LEVELS OF INTRODUCTORY CLINICAL FUNCTIONING

Ideally, this book is intended for all speech-language pathology students before entering the first clinical practicum experience. It can also be used simultaneously, but this will not enable you to get a head start on the clinical process. For many of you, this first clinical experience will occur on the undergraduate level, but for others, it will be undertaken at the graduate level. Your status, undergraduate or graduate, does not have any bearing on using this book, as it addresses clinical problems that cut across all skill levels. The focus is on persistent clinical problems that nearly all students encounter. These ongoing clinical problems may stand in your way of achieving clinical competence unless they are understood and dealt with in a forthright and professional fashion.

The actual clinical problems that you encounter may differ somewhat, depending on your place in the learning process. This can be compared with the well-known parable of how a number of blind or partially sighted persons describe an elephant. An individual's description can only be based on the part of the elephant that is under exploration, and this will be influenced by the degree of visual challenge. Problems you may see will vary according to your involvement in the discovery process and your understanding of the problem.

In general, the nature of the clinical problems you may encounter could differ as you move through three stages: (1) immediately prior to starting the clinical experience, (2) becoming initially involved with the clinical experience, and (3) being actively involved in the clinical experience. Clinicians in the third stage will already have an initial evaluation in place (done either by oneself or another), will have had long- and short-range objectives approved by their supervisors, and will be in the process of designing and executing therapy.

Conceptually, the "ideal case" for your passage from the undergraduate classroom to clinic, or from the graduate classroom to clinic for graduate students without any previous clinical experience, can be represented by Figure I–1. This smooth transition is rarely seen in practice because movement across the three stages is not strictly sequential.

Some behaviors and skills will not be acquired by you at the time they are expected to be developed. Movement back and forth, pendulum fashion, is the rule rather than the exception. Figure I–2 better reflects the passage experienced by most of you. Overlap in process, the need to learn what should have been already acquired or, in the worst case, to relearn material, is represented in this figure. If you are a graduate student, the model (and the problems at each stage) remain the same, but your expectations and those of your supervisors and professors will be different.

STAGE ONE: IMMEDIATELY PRIOR TO STARTING THE CLINICAL EXPERIENCE

Many students about to enter the first clinical experience have admitted to me that they were "scared to death" about their upcoming transition into the clinic. This mind-set is counterproductive because this transition can be exhilarating and can often make or break their career. To understand these feelings better, I once

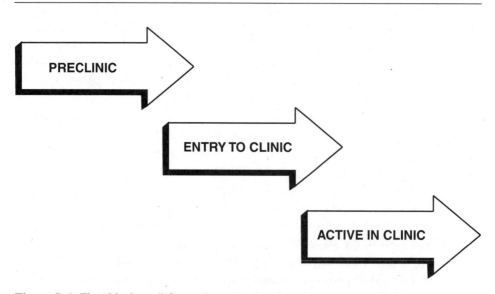

Figure I–1 The "ideal case" for students moving from classroom to clinic.

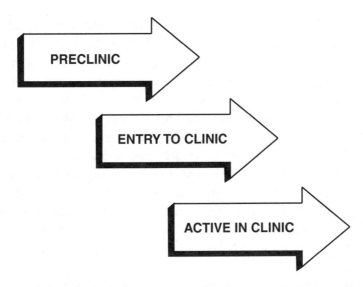

Figure I–2 The typical experience for students moving from classroom to clinic.

developed an entrance survey that was completed by students about to enter their first clinical practicum. These students were asked to write their feelings, attitudes, and perceptions of their upcoming experience. The impact of the impending professional experience was clarified after reviewing these data. In sum, the survey revealed that the students perceived a disjunction between the classroom and the clinic and also a discontinuity between the knowledge they had and the knowledge that they believed was needed to perform successfully in the clinical situation. These students did not know how the clinic and the classroom were related or whether their knowledge base was sufficient.

On the basis of the survey results, it was determined that the biggest problem for beginning students was the preponderance of negative feelings. In their descriptions, words such as "anxious," "nervousness," "uneasy," "uncomfortable," "fright," "scared," "overwhelmed," "intense frustration," "apprehension," "paranoia," and "worried" were plentiful. Chan, Carter, and McAllister (1994) state that

> anxiety appears to have an impact on the nature and quality of students' clinical learning experiences. Therefore, identification of both the level of anxiety experienced and the factors contributing significantly to the anxiety may facilitate constructive modification of the clinical learning experience. (p. 126)

It is hoped that this book will help reduce your anxiety by preparing you for your clinical experience.

In addition, some of your predecessors believed that they were not academically prepared to undergo involvement with the clinical process, and other beginning clinicians questioned their overall competence. Positive descriptors, although occasionally present, were infrequent. It appears that it is necessary to bridge the gap between the classroom and clinic in both an experiential and intellectual fashion to (1) help in the status change from students to professionals, and (2) give guidance on how to help translate classroom materials into practical tools. If, in making these transitions, you do not have convenient access to your supervisor at some times, you will need somewhere to turn for assistance. In such cases, let this book perform this function. You will find leafing through this entire book to be helpful, as it will enable you to prepare for what is expected of you.

STAGE TWO: BECOMING INVOLVED WITH THE CLINICAL EXPERIENCE

Beginning clinical students frequently get bogged down with paperwork. My previous students repeatedly cited paperwork as being the number one problem encountered during this phase of their clinical process. Haynes and Hartman (1975) clearly address this problem in their assessment of the paperwork agony. They state

> In our training institutions, beginning speech clinicians are required to write several types of clinical reports (diagnostic, initial, progress, final, etc.). It has been the experience of the present authors, both as students and as supervisors, that these reports are a major source of conflict, negative emotion and student insecurity. Each quarter in universities across the country, there exists a massive ebb and flow of clinical reports between supervisors and student clinicians. The reports are submitted to the supervisors and then returned to the students with numerous multicolored criticisms. These flaws must then be corrected and the reports resubmitted to the supervisor for further scrutiny. So it goes, back and forth. In many cases, the report goes through this process so repeatedly that the finished product is almost totally written in installments by the supervisor. The reasons behind the supervisor's manifold revisions are not always clear to the burgeoning speech clinician, however, these students are assured that they will understand the rationale and substance of the corrections when they have had more experience with report writing. (p. 7)

It is obvious that if the ambiguity and confusion can be removed from the paperwork process, you will avoid undue anxiety and your time and energy can be better channeled, enabling you to be more productive. Further, by reducing some of the mystery of how you should approach various aspects of the paperwork process, you can develop more positive feelings about your performance earlier in the clinical experience—ultimately achieving more success. An increase in the quality of your therapy should be observed as you are freed from the burdens of paperwork.

STAGE THREE: BEING ACTIVELY INVOLVED IN THE CLINICAL EXPERIENCE

This group is knowledgeable in therapeutic techniques taught in the classroom, but not in the actual orchestration of the therapy session or therapeutic process. This is the major clinical problem for this group. Most of this orchestration is learned through actual experience, trial and error, and feedback from your supervisor's evaluations. If, however, many of these aspects can be presented, explained, and demonstrated before you are expected to conduct therapy, you will not be as frustrated as you struggle with understanding what a therapy session is all about. Clients will benefit because their sessions will flow more smoothly and therapy will be more effective and efficient. Supervisors will also benefit because their time can be spent helping you master the more important advanced aspects of the therapeutic process. The gains are far reaching.

HOW TO USE THIS BOOK

You will use this book differently depending on which of the three groups best represents your status. Generally, because not all of you experience the transition into the clinic in the same way, this book could not be strictly organized to fit the "ideal type" shown in Figure I-1. The best advice is for you to read the entire book to determine the most relevant material to you at that particular time and to note mentally what additional information is included for future reference. Later, this book will become a resource to assist navigating within a new stage. To assist in this endeavor, the following comments apply.

The first group, those of you about to start the clinical experience, should begin reading this book about one month prior to your actual involvement in clinical practicum. It is during this time frame that you have the most anxiety. By reading this book and obtaining information about the clinical process, as well as becoming knowledgeable about the expectations, anxiety levels should decline. The result is a more positive mind-set, which can only help you get started on the right foot.

Remarkably, when you actively prepare for your clinical practicum, you develop a "stake" in the outcome. This softens the perceived disjunction between the classroom and clinic and between acquired knowledge and the knowledge you believe is needed.

The second group, those of you getting involved with the clinical experience, will use this book to help you survive the voluminous amount of required paperwork. It would be in your best interest to implement the system offered in chapter 6 to organize and manage this mountain of paper, paper, and more paper. At this point in your professional training, this book will be your constant companion when writing evaluations, lesson plans, and progress notes. This book will also be the source used to obtain information about maintaining records during therapy sessions. Nothing puts a chill on student enthusiasm so effectively as that first paperwork "snowstorm." To help you survive this phase, chapters 1 through 6 will be particularly helpful.

This book will also be helpful to those of you actively involved in the clinical experience (the third group). You will need help orchestrating therapy sessions as you come to terms with the therapeutic process. You will find the chapter dealing with therapy suggestions (chapter 7) most helpful. You will probably find that these pages will rapidly become worn. Avoiding the problems presented in this chapter and implementing the solutions provided will help you function more effectively and efficiently. You will also find the information in chapter 8 on self-evaluation pertinent to this level of functioning.

When discussing how to use this book, it is necessary to comment about performance proficiency. Functioning is cumulative. If you are in the third group and are having difficulty writing behavioral objectives or evaluations or both, you will have to acquire these skills just as would a student in the second group. You will consult chapters 1 and 2 to help brush up on behavioral objectives, and you will consult chapters 3 and 4 to assist with writing evaluations. You will rely on this book to refresh and renew your performance skills. You need to realize, however, that skills might not improve by jumping ahead and trying to incorporate material or skills that are best left to higher levels of involvement in clinical functioning. Remember: Trying to do too much too soon might lead to a failure to learn the basics and might unnecessarily negate performance for otherwise good students. Instead, this book should be used as a preview of what is expected as you mentally role-play your part as more advanced clinical students soon to be professionals. Those of you who want to succeed will do this anyway, but all of you will benefit by using mental role-playing.

CONCLUSION

Bridging the gap in knowledge between the classroom and clinic is possible. This is something that cannot be done solely in the classroom or in the clinic. You can and should use the transition time between the two settings to prepare yourself better for your upcoming experience. If you are provided with direction, you can actively attempt to bridge this gap. Previously, it often appeared that students were expected to learn effective and efficient clinical performance through trial and error; however, a better approach is possible. It is far more logical and supportive of effective teaching techniques if these common faux pas are identified so that they can be counteracted or prevented. There is no reason why you should make the same mistakes as yesterday's beginning clinicians. If these clinical problem areas are identified and addressed, many of these inappropriate clinical behaviors will be eliminated and more effective clinical performance will result. This is the intent of this book. This book is the tool that you can use to help yourself bridge the gap and take the first step toward achieving professional status. The end result should be that your clinical performance starts at a higher level and far surpasses that of those previous beginning clinicians who did not have access to this tool and of current beginning clinicians who chose not to use this tool.

Returning to the elephant parable, it is apparent that an adequate description of an elephant cannot be obtained through exploration of single or isolated parts. Likewise, with the clinical experience. To take those first steps toward achieving professional status, integration of all parts of the clinical experience is necessary. It is necessary to have positive feelings toward the clinical experience, mastery as well as expedient execution of all parts of the paperwork process, and knowledge about, as well as appropriate application of, clinical information in the orchestration of therapy sessions.

If you are conscientious and try to prepare yourself for each step of the clinical process before actually taking that step, common clinical errors should be prevented. Your supervisor will thus not have to deal with minor aspects of the clinical process and will be able to direct his or her energy toward helping you achieve a higher level of performance than was previously possible.

This introduction is a bridge between the stated intent of the preface and the much more specific content of chapters 1 through 8. It is, therefore, quite short. It is the author's earnest hope that your travels across your bridges to becoming a competent professional will also be short.

KNOW IT! USE IT!

Upon reading this introduction, you should be able to:

1. state 10 words describing feelings, attitudes, and/or perceptions frequently encountered in the "immediately prior to starting the clinical experience" stage
2. state the number one problem encountered when in the "becoming involved with the clinical experience" stage
3. state the major clinical problem when in the "being actively involved in the clinical experience" stage
4. state the single most important way this book can be used in each of the three clinical stages

REFERENCES

Chan, J., Carter, S., & McAllister, L. (1994). Sources of anxiety related to clinical education in speech-language pathology students. In M. Bruce (Ed.), *Proceedings of the 1994 International & Interdisciplinary Conference on Clinical Supervision: Toward the 21st century* (pp. 126–132). Houston, TX: University of Houston.

Haynes, W., & Hartman, D. (1975). The agony of report writing: A new look at an old problem. *The Journal of the National Student Speech and Hearing Association, 3,* 7–15.

CHAPTER 1

Behavioral Objectives: Background

CHAPTER HIGHLIGHTS

- *background information on behavioral objectives*
- *reasons for writing behavioral objectives*
- *composition of behavioral objectives*
- *construction of behavioral objectives*
- *application of behavioral objectives*
- *the role of behavioral objectives in lesson plans*

Robert Mager (1984) is responsible for the early work on instructional or behavioral objectives. Later, Donald Mowrer (1988) expanded Mager's ideas and applied them to speech-language pathology. Mager defined an objective as "a description of a performance you want learners to be able to exhibit before you consider them competent" (p. 5). Mowrer adopted a more research-oriented definition when he defined a behavioral objective as one "which is stated in terms of behaviors which can be observed and measured" (p. 148). According to Mager, objectives are important for three reasons, as follows.

First, Mager said that when objectives are not clearly defined, one does not have a good basis for selecting materials, content, or procedures (p. 5). In other words, if you do not know where you are headed in terms of the remediation process, it is impossible to design or implement a therapy program to help a client succeed. Clinicians and clients alike function in a state of confusion if it is not known what the client is expected to accomplish as a result of the therapeutic process.

A second reason for clearly stating objectives is to determine whether they have been accomplished (p. 5). It is only possible to assess the client's success formally or informally if both parties (the client and clinician) know the desired end result. In other words, if clinicians do not know what they are working toward, they will not know when the objective has been reached.

A third reason for stating objectives is to enable the client to participate meaningfully (p. 6). What a client is expected to learn is not supposed to be kept secret. It is not possible for a client to cooperate fully if he is oblivious to the nature of the task and its accomplishment.

Beginning clinicians need to write clear behavioral objectives as a step toward ensuring effective therapy. To write these objectives, you must look beyond the client's obvious problem(s) and analyze all data that have been collected during formal and informal assessments, synthesize those data, and formulate an informed opinion. Objectives are better when you have determined the client's current level of functioning and the level at which the client should be functioning. This allows you to formulate the steps for enabling the client to move from where he is functioning to where he should be functioning. Objectives must therefore reflect the emphases of the therapy program or they will never become the base for any meaningful therapy program.

COMPONENTS OF A BEHAVIORAL OBJECTIVE

For a behavioral objective to be meaningful, the primary reader's (at first, this will be your clinical supervisor) understanding of a client's performance must be identical with that of the writer's (in this case, you, the beginning clinician). If these interpretations are not identical, the objective is not well written and misinterpretation results. If this is the case, objectives need to be revised to convey the correct intent. When your goal is to write meaningful behavioral objectives, you must include three components: performance, condition, and criterion. Each of these is discussed in turn.

Performance Component

Mager (1984) has noted that an objective must state what a learner is expected to do or perform in order to demonstrate mastery of the objective. The little word "DO" is the key here, as an objective cannot be complete without the "doing" aspect being included. Mager suggested that the question "What is the learner DOING when demonstrating achievement of the objective?" (p. 25) be asked to check whether the objective includes performance. To assess whether performance is addressed, Mowrer (1988) urges that the question "Can I count it?" be used (p. 158). He also says that one of the major pitfalls in writing the performance component of behavioral objectives is the use of ill-defined or vague verbs. Mager also cautioned against using "slippery" verbs such as *know, understand,* and *appreciate* that can be interpreted in many ways (p. 20). Others in the field (Wheeler & Fox, 1977) have also cautioned against using ambiguous action verbs such as *demonstrate, perform,* and *select* (p. 26). You need to know that the performance aspect of the behavioral objective is the "verb" component (Mowrer, 1988, p. 160). Exhibit 1–1 lists acceptable verbs for use in objectives.

Exhibit 1–2 presents a list of verbs to be avoided. Because many supervisors in speech-language pathology accept the verb "use" (it is, after all, a natural aspect of performance), I recommend you discuss its acceptability with your supervisor. Before you do, give some thought to both sides of the question and see how, or why, the verb is either appropriate or inappropriate.

Overt and Covert Verbs

Mager (1984) differentiated between types of verbs used in behavioral objectives. According to him, overt verbs refer to performance that is directly observable. This type of performance can be observed through either vision or audition. Covert verbs refer to performance that cannot be directly observed. This type of performance "is mental, invisible, cognitive or internal" (p. 43). Covert performance can only be detected if the client is asked to say or do something (p. 43). Some examples of covert verbs are *discriminate, recall, identify,* and *solve.*

Covert performance can only be correctly stated in a behavioral objective if there is a direct way of determining whether the objective has been satisfied.

Exhibit 1–1 Acceptable Verbs

build	match	repeat
compare	name	repeat orally
construct	place	say
contrast	point	smile
count	pour	sort
demand	press lever	state
diagram	put	tell what
draw	reach	walk
fold	read orally	write
label	recite	
list	remove	

Source: Data from R.F. Mager, 1984, D.E. Mowrer, 1988, and A.H. Wheeler and L. Fox, 1977.

Exhibit 1–2 Verbs to Avoid

acknowledge	enjoy	like
acquaint	familiarize	make
apply	feel	plan
appreciate	give	play
arrange	grasp the significance	realize
believe	of	respond to
communicate	have faith in	select
demonstrate	internalize	understand
develop	know	use
discover	learn	

Source: Data from R.F. Mager, 1984, D.E. Mowrer, 1988, and A.H. Wheeler and L. Fox, 1977.

Mager's rule is, "Whenever the performance stated in an objective is covert, add an indicator behavior to the objective" (1984, p. 44). Some of Mager's (1984, p. 44) examples showing measurable indicator behavior are:

[1.] be able to add numbers (write the solutions) written in binary notation

[2.] be able to identify (underline or circle) misspelled words on a given page of news copy

Wheeler and Fox (1977) list action verbs that are not directly observable and "should not be used when writing instructional objectives" (p. 27). A few examples of these action verbs are *recognize, infer, analyze,* and *know.* According to Mager (1984), however, these verbs can be used if an indicator behavior is included. Some of the verbs on Wheeler and Fox's list are shown in Exhibit 1–3.

Performance Examples Common to Speech-Language Pathology

In this section, the performance portion of behavioral objectives is addressed by providing pertinent examples of some of the commonly encountered communication disorders and problem behaviors. For ease of reference, examples are given in the following order throughout this chapter: articulation, phonology, language, voice, fluency, pragmatics, and problem behavior. This order will be adopted for consistency.

Performance Examples 1: Articulation
• correctly produce the /r/ phoneme

Exhibit 1–3 Action Verbs Requiring Indicators

analyze	deduce	realize fully
be aware	determine	recognize
become competent	discriminate	solve
be curious	distinguish	test
concentrate	generate	think
conclude	infer	think critically
create	perceive	wonder

Note: Examples of both overt and covert verbs can be found in the "Performance Examples Common to Speech-Language Pathology" section in this chapter. If the above-listed verbs or similar verbs appear in the performance component, the verbs are covert and indicator behaviors must be added.

Source: Data from A.H. Wheeler and W.L. Fox, 1977.

- correctly imitate /s/
- raise his tongue tip to the alveolar ridge
- auditorially discriminate (by raising his hand) /s/ from /f/
- correctly monitor (state if correct or not) production of the /l/ phoneme
- correctly monitor (self-correct) production of the /s/ phoneme

Performance Examples 2: Phonology
- close syllables
- correctly imitate the consonant clusters /sk/, /sp/, and /st/
- produce both stressed and unstressed syllables
- produce voiceless consonants
- produce fricatives or affricates
- produce liquids

Performance Examples 3: Language
- name pictures spontaneously
- identify (name) pictures expressively
- identify (point to) pictures receptively
- use present progressive tense correctly
- use the pronouns "he" and "she" appropriately
- use plurals correctly

- use correct subject-verb agreement
- follow directions
- use the prepositions "in" and "on" correctly
- use three-word utterances
- ask questions
- say complete sentences

Performance Examples 4: Voice
- identify (by raising his hand) vocal abuses
- explain laryngeal functioning
- use appropriate pitch
- produce easy onset of voice
- produce appropriate oral resonance

Performance Examples 5: Fluency
- identify (by saying "there") nonfluencies
- read fluently
- speak fluently
- cancel stuttering episodes
- identify (state) factors in his stuttering equation
- use pull-outs

Performance Examples 6: Pragmatics
- request (by pointing or using eye gaze) an object
- take turns
- attend to (look at) the speaker
- initiate a greeting
- specify a topic
- maintain a topic

Performance Examples 7: Problem Behavior
- walk into the therapy room
- sit without kicking
- attend to (look at) a picture when directed
- answer questions about a story
- perform tasks
- follow directions

> **QUICK CHECK**
>
> You must critically examine your behavioral objectives to make certain a performance aspect has been included. If it has, check to see whether the verb is overt or covert. If the verb is covert, a behavior indicator is needed. If the desired behavior is not immediately apparent, the objective is not written clearly. In this case, it is necessary to rethink *exactly* what the client is supposed to do and then rewrite the objective until there is no ambiguity regarding the client's role.

Condition Component

The second aspect to be included in a well-written behavioral objective is the condition under which the performance is to be done. These are the conditions that will be imposed on clients when they are demonstrating their achievement of an objective. Mager (1984) stated that the definition of terminal behavior should be "detailed enough to be sure the desired performance would be recognized by another competent person, and detailed enough so that others understand your intent as YOU understand it" (p. 51). Mowrer (1988) stated:

> Conditions specify what you will provide to the individual in order to help him do the task, or they may describe what you will deny the learner. They can also pinpoint where the behavior will be performed, when it will be performed, and in whose presence it will be performed. (p. 160)

Mowrer (1988) further added that because conditions describe the situation in which the behavior is to be performed, it comprises the "adjective" portion of the objective (p. 160). Some examples of conditions as stated by Mager (1984, p. 50) are:

- Given a problem of the following type . . .
- Given a list of . . .
- Given any reference of the learner's choice . . .
- Without the aid of references . . .
- Without the aid of a slide rule . . .
- Without the aid of tools . . .

Mager (1984, p. 51) provides the following four questions to use as a guide to identify important aspects of target or terminal performances:

1. What will the learner be allowed to use?
2. What will the learner be denied?
3. Under what conditions will you expect the desired performance to occur?
4. Are there any skills that you are specifically NOT trying to develop? Does the objective exclude such skills?

It is not obligatory for behavioral objectives to contain a condition aspect. If the objective is clearly stated without it, a condition is not necessary. If someone else's interpretation does not match yours, then further description is needed. Add as much description as necessary to communicate the intent to others clearly (Mager, 1984, pp. 68, 69).

Condition Examples Common to Speech-Language Pathology

Examples of conditions included in behavioral objectives for some of the major communication disorders and problem behavior will now be given in the order used for the performance component.

Condition Examples 1: Articulation
- in all word positions
- in isolation
- with his mouth opened at least 1½ inches
- in consonant-vowel combinations
- during spontaneous conversation
- during reading
- without a model

Condition Examples 2: Phonology
- on spontaneously produced monosyllabic target words
- without a pause between the two consonants
- in bisyllabic words
- when preceding vowels
- of all appropriate contexts

Condition Examples 3: Language
- in a children's dictionary
- of common objects
- given a field of three
- while describing pictures
- during conversation

- in a structured situation
- when telling a story
- in less than 5 seconds
- when describing spatial relations
- without prompts
- beginning with "how"
- using the conjunction "and"

Condition Examples 4: Voice
- when eight choices are presented
- one session after the clinician's explanation
- while producing /ɑ/
- on the vowels /o/ and /i/
- on vowel-consonant combinations
- on vowels

Condition Examples 5: Fluency
- consisting of prolongations lasting longer than 2 seconds
- in front of his class
- for 5 minutes
- while talking on the telephone
- the session after this discussion occurred
- while speaking to the principal

Condition Examples 6: Pragmatics
- which is out of reach
- when a familiar joint action routine is initiated by a significant other
- during communication episodes
- upon seeing the clinician
- during each therapy session
- initiated by someone else

Condition Examples 7: Problem Behavior
- without yanking the clinician's arm
- after the removal of restraints
- when a desirable toy is within reaching distance
- without throwing a temper tantrum
- within a 2-second period

QUICK CHECK

If a condition aspect is needed in a particular behavioral objective, it must be written specifically to avoid misunderstanding. If the condition is not written specifically, a mismatch may occur between the writer's (your) intent and the reader's (your supervisor's) interpretation.

Criterion Component

The third component to be included in behavioral objectives is criterion that states how well the learner is expected to perform. Mager says that "a criterion is the standard by which performance is evaluated, the yardstick by which achievement of the objective is assessed" (p. 71). In this manner, it can be determined whether the therapy techniques were successful in accomplishing the behavioral objectives. The desired criterion can be specified in several ways. According to Mowrer (1988), "the criterion resembles an 'adverb' statement in that it states how or when the objective is to be met. It could also be considered an adjective statement because often the criterion consists of a description of 'how many behaviors'" (p.161). Mager (p. 78) stated that often the criterion is set by answering the following questions:

1. How well must a student be able to perform in order for practice to be the only requirement for improvement?
2. How competent must the student be in order to be ready for the next assignment (the next objective, the next course, the job itself)?

For Mager (1984), criterion is frequently stated in terms of speed, accuracy, and quality. In the speech-language pathology discipline, accuracy is frequently cited. Speed is cited less frequently and quality is rarely cited. These three parameters are briefly discussed here.

A common way to describe performance relative to speed "is to describe a time limit within which a given performance must occur" (Mager, 1984, p. 74). An example cited by Mager is *"four of five malfunctions must be located within ten minutes each"* (1984, p. 75, emphasis in original). Accuracy is another way to measure criterion. Some of Mager's (p. 79) examples are:

- and solutions must be accurate to the nearest whole number
- with materials weighed accurately to the nearest gram

- correct to at least three significant figures
- with no more than two incorrect entries for every ten pages of log
- with the listening accurate enough so that no more than one request for repeated information is made for each customer contact

Quality is another way to measure criterion. To communicate the desired quality of performance, the amount of acceptable deviation from perfection or another standard would have to be defined (Mager, 1984, p. 83). One of Mager's examples is to "be able to adjust the PPI [round TV screen in a missile] range-marker to acceptable roundness . . . [defined as] no more than one-eighth inch deviation from a standard template" (p. 83). Fortunately, similar criteria are rare in speech-language pathology.

Criterion Examples Common to Speech-Language Pathology

The following examples are not divided into accuracy, speed, and quality because these criteria are not equally distributed across behavioral objectives written in speech-language pathology. It is also unnecessary to cite examples by type of communication disorders or problem behavior because these examples are not specific as to type of disorder. This will be clear upon reviewing the list.

Criterion Examples
- in 90% of his attempts
- in 90% of all appropriate contexts
- in 8 of 10 attempts
- on 8 of 10 trials
- in 20 of 25 pictures
- with 90% agreement
- with less than 0.5 stuttered words per minute
- in two of the three weekly therapy sessions
- for 25 minutes
- five new words
- twice during a 10-minute time segment
- three consecutive trials

A criterion of 90% is usually used in speech-language pathology. In certain situations (mentally challenged, extremely young, and so on), however, a criterion of 80% is frequently used.

QUICK CHECK

If a criterion is not specified, the objective is not complete. Without a criterion, it is not possible to determine whether the objective has been accomplished.

SAMPLES OF WELL-WRITTEN BEHAVIORAL OBJECTIVES

At this point, you should be able to state the three components of a behavioral objective, describe each component, divide an objective into the components, and give pertinent examples. You will now have an opportunity to check your mastery. This can be done in two ways. The first way involves looking at the following sample objectives and following the text. The second way involves skipping pages beginning with the ensuing *Sample Objectives* section and continuing up to the *Application and Importance of Behavioral Objectives* section, completing the worksheets found in Appendix 1–A, and then checking your responses with the worksheets found in Appendix 1–B. If this is your choice, please turn to Appendix 1–A at this time. If you have selected the first option, the emphasis will be placed on reviewing examples of behavioral objectives that include these three components. Behavioral objectives relevant to some of the major types of communication disorders as well as problem behavior are given. Although many formats are available to "lead in" to behavioral objectives, the phrase, "The client will . . ." is understood for all examples in this section. If you have selected the first option, read on.

Sample Objectives 1: Articulation
1. correctly produce the /r/ phoneme in all positions of words in 90% of his attempts
2. correctly imitate /s/ in isolation in 8 of 10 attempts
3. raise his tongue tip to the alveolar ridge with his mouth opened at least $1\frac{1}{2}$ inches on 8 of 10 trials
4. auditorially discriminate (by raising his hand) /s/ from /f/ in consonant–vowel combinations in 90% of his attempts
5. correctly monitor (state if correct or not) production of the /l/ phoneme during spontaneous conversation in 90% of his attempts
6. correctly monitor (self-correct) 90% of the incorrect /s/ productions during reading

If it is difficult to separate these objectives into the components of performance, condition, and criterion, it would be wise to go back and review the pertinent sections before continuing. Every component included in these objectives has previously appeared in this chapter.

The following numbers correspond to the behavioral objectives just listed. The *performance* aspect of each objective is:

1. correctly produce the /r/ phoneme
2. correctly imitate /s/
3. raise his tongue tip to the alveolar ridge
4. auditorially discriminate (by raising his hand) /s/ from /f/
5. correctly monitor (state if correct or not) production of the /l/ phoneme
6. correctly monitor (self-correct) incorrect /s/ productions

The following *conditions* are present in the behavioral objectives:

1. in all positions of words
2. in isolation
3. with his mouth opened at least 1½ inches
4. in consonant–vowel combinations
5. during spontaneous conversation
6. during reading

The *criterion* for each of the behavioral objectives is:

1. in 90% of his attempts
2. in 8 of 10 attempts
3. on 8 of 10 trials
4. in 90% of his attempts
5. in 90% of his attempts
6. 90%

Sample Objectives 2: Phonology

1. close syllables on spontaneously produced monosyllabic target words in 90% of his attempts (Note: This objective addresses the process deletion of final consonants.)
2. correctly imitate the consonant clusters /sk/, /sp/, and /st/ without a pause between the two consonants in 90% of his attempts (Note: This objective addresses the process cluster reduction.)

3. produce unstressed syllables in bisyllabic words in 90% of his attempts. (Note: This objective addresses the process deletion of unstressed syllables.)
4. produce voiceless consonants when preceding vowels in 90% of the appropriate contexts (Note: This objective addresses the process prevocalic voicing of consonants.)
5. produce fricatives or affricates in 90% of the appropriate contexts (Note: This objective addresses the process stopping.)
6. produce liquids in 90% of the appropriate contexts (Note: This objective addresses the process gliding.)

The numbers that follow correspond to the behavioral objectives just listed. The *performance* aspect of each objective is:

1. close syllables
2. correctly imitate the consonant clusters /sk/, /sp/, and /st/
3. produce unstressed syllables
4. produce voiceless consonants
5. produce fricatives or affricates
6. produce liquids

The following *conditions* are present in the behavioral objectives:

1. on spontaneously produced monosyllabic target words
2. without a pause between the two consonants
3. in bisyllabic words
4. when preceding vowels
5. the appropriate contexts
6. the appropriate contexts

The *criterion* for each of the behavioral objectives is:

1. in 90% of his attempts
2. in 90% of his attempts
3. in 90% of his attempts
4. in 90% of the appropriate contexts
5. 90%
6. 90%

Sample Objectives 3: Language
1. spontaneously name 20 of 25 pictures in a children's dictionary

2. expressively identify (name) pictures of common objects in 90% of his attempts
3. receptively identify (point to) pictures given in a field of three in 8 of 10 attempts
4. correctly use present progressive tense while describing 20 of 25 pictures that are not visible to the clinician
5. appropriately use the pronouns "he" and "she" during conversation in 90% of his attempts
6. correctly use regular plurals in at least 90% of his attempts while telling a story

The following *performance* aspects can be found in the behavioral objectives just listed:

1. spontaneously name pictures
2. expressively identify (name) pictures
3. receptively identify (point to) pictures
4. correctly use present progressive tense
5. appropriately use the pronouns "he" and "she"
6. correctly use regular plurals

The following *conditions* are included in the behavioral objectives:

1. in a children's dictionary
2. of common objects
3. given in a field of three
4. while describing pictures that are not visible to the clinician
5. during conversation
6. while telling a story

The *criterion* contained in each of the behavioral objectives is:

1. 20 of 25
2. in 90% of his attempts
3. in 8 of 10 attempts
4. 20 of 25
5. in 90% of his attempts
6. in at least 90% of his attempts

Sample Objectives 4: Voice
1. identify (by raising his hand) at least seven of his vocal abuses when all possible abuses are stated

2. explain three steps in laryngeal functioning one session after the clinician's explanation
3. use appropriate pitch while producing /ɑ/ in 8 of 10 trials
4. produce easy onset of voice on the vowels /o/ and /i/ in 90% of his attempts
5. produce appropriate oral resonance on vowel–consonant combinations in 90% of his attempts

The following *performance* aspects can be identified in the objectives just listed:

1. identify (by raising his hand) vocal abuses
2. explain steps in laryngeal functioning
3. use appropriate pitch
4. produce easy onset of voice
5. produce appropriate oral resonance

The following *conditions* are present in the behavioral objectives:

1. when all possible abuses are stated
2. one session after the clinician's explanation
3. while producing /ɑ/
4. on the vowels /o/ and /i/
5. on vowel–consonant combinations

The *criterion* for each of the behavioral objectives is:

1. at least seven
2. three
3. in 8 of 10 trials
4. in 90% of his attempts
5. in 90% of his attempts

Sample Objectives 5: Fluency

1. identify (by saying "there") 90% of his nonfluencies that consist of prolongations lasting longer than 2 seconds
2. read in front of his class with less than 0.5 stuttered words per minute
3. speak with less than 0.5 stuttered words per minute during 5 minutes of spontaneous conversation with the clinician
4. cancel 90% of the stuttering episodes that occur while talking on the telephone
5. identify (state) all factors in his stuttering equation one session after this discussion occurred

6. use pull-outs during all episodes of blocking while speaking to the principal for 5 minutes

The following *performance* aspects are included in the behavioral objectives just listed:

1. identify (by saying "there") his nonfluencies
2. read
3. speak
4. cancel stuttering episodes
5. identify (state) factors in his stuttering equation
6. use pull-outs during episodes of blocking

Conditions found in the behavioral objectives are:

1. that consist of prolongations lasting longer than 2 seconds
2. in front of his class
3. during 5 minutes of spontaneous conversation with the clinician
4. that occur while talking on the telephone
5. one session after this discussion occurred
6. while speaking to the principal for 5 minutes

Note that confusion can result in interpreting the third and sixth behavioral objectives. A tendency exists to include automatically "numbers" as the criterion or as a part of the criteria. This is not always correct. Therefore you must exert caution. The phrase "5 minutes" in both the third and sixth objective is part of the condition component and not the criterion.

The *criterion* contained in each of the behavioral objectives is:

1. 90% of his nonfluencies
2. with less than 0.5 stuttered words per minute
3. with less than 0.5 stuttered words per minute
4. 90%
5. all [implies 100%]
6. all [implies 100%]

Sample Objectives 6: Pragmatics

1. request (by pointing or using eye gaze) an object that is out of reach twice during a 10-minute time segment

2. take three consecutive turns when a familiar joint action routine is initiated by a significant other
3. attend to (look at) the speaker during two of three communication episodes
4. initiate a greeting upon seeing the clinician on four of five appropriate occasions
5. specify a topic once during each therapy session
6. maintain a topic initiated by someone else for three conversational turns

The following *performance* aspects can be found in the behavioral objectives just listed:

1. request (by pointing or using eye gaze) an object
2. take consecutive turns
3. attend to (look at) the speaker
4. initiate a greeting
5. specify a topic
6. maintain a topic

The behavioral objectives include the following *conditions*:

1. that is out of reach
2. when a familiar joint action routine is initiated by a significant other
3. during communication episodes
4. upon seeing the clinician
5. during each therapy session
6. initiated by someone else

The following *criteria* are contained in the behavioral objectives:

1. twice during a 10-minute time segment
2. three
3. two of three
4. on four of five appropriate occasions
5. once
6. for three conversational turns

Sample Objectives 7: Problem Behavior
1. walk into the therapy room without yanking the clinician's arm in two of the three weekly therapy sessions
2. sit without kicking for 5 minutes after the removal of restraints [your hands on the client's knees]

3. attend to (look at) a picture for 2 minutes when a desirable toy is within reaching distance
4. perform a specified task for 25 minutes without throwing a temper tantrum
5. follow 8 of 10 directions within 2 seconds of the initial presentation

The following *performances* can be identified in the behavioral objectives just listed:

1. walk into the therapy room
2. sit without kicking
3. attend to (look at) a picture
4. perform a specified task
5. follow directions

The following *conditions* can be identified in the behavioral objectives:

1. without yanking the clinician's arm
2. after the removal of restraints [Note: your hands on the client's knees]
3. when a desirable toy is within reaching distance
4. without throwing a temper tantrum
5. within 2 seconds of the initial presentation

The following *criteria* are contained in the behavioral objectives:

1. in two of the three weekly therapy sessions
2. for 5 minutes
3. for 2 minutes
4. for 25 minutes
5. 8 of 10

APPLICATION AND IMPORTANCE OF BEHAVIORAL OBJECTIVES

The process of being able to understand and write behavioral objectives has far-reaching ramifications in speech-language pathology. Mowrer (1988) stated, "Behavioral objectives are included as a basic ingredient of many commercially developed instructional programs available to speech clinicians" (p. 149). Therefore, if you do not understand behavioral objectives, it will be difficult to conduct the programs and obtain and record responses in the intended manner. Mowrer (1988) also stated, "Most federal grant applications which pertain to any form of instruction require that objectives be clearly indicated and tied to performance measures" (p. 149). Although grant-writing is not foremost at this point in your career, it may become important in the not-too-distant future. With the practice in writing behavioral objectives that is gained during clinical practicum, basic skills are learned that can easily be applied to the grant-writing process. There are more-immediate reasons for gaining expertise in writing behavioral objectives.

Lesson Plans

Behavioral objectives comprise a major part of lesson plans (also referred to as pretherapy plans or clinical strategy outlines). Before entering each therapy session, a lesson plan, which consists of realistic goals to be accomplished during that session, must be developed. These goals are written in the form of behavioral objectives. Lesson plans can be developed for each session separately or for all sessions held within a week. Factors to be considered when determining the frequency with which lesson plans are written are the length of the sessions, the frequency of the sessions, and the client's progress. If progress is fast, a new plan should be devised for each session. If progress is slow, a weekly plan may be adequate. Lesson plans are usually divided into two main parts. The first part consists of session objectives that are called short-term objectives, short-range objectives, lesson objectives, subobjectives, or transitional objectives. Regardless of the terminology used, they are all expressed in behavioral objectives.

Short-Range Objectives

According to Thompson (1977), "Short-term objectives are concerned with small units of behavior and should be attainable in a short time" (p. 54). Thompson also said, "The short-term objectives identify the appropriate activities through which the child will progress toward the expectancies stated in the long-term plan" (p. 6). Silverman (1984) stated, "Short-term goals specify abilities that clients must acquire before they can achieve long-term goals" (p. 230).

The second part of a lesson plan consists of procedures used to meet each objective listed. Additional requirements for lesson plans vary from training program to training program. It is quite probable that you will be required to provide a written rationale for each objective.

A lesson plan for a child aged 10 years, 3 months can be found in Exhibit 1–4. It includes short-term objectives and procedures for a mild articulation problem.

Long-Range Objectives

Long-range objectives, which are written in behavioral objective style, are also known as long-term objectives or long-term goals and might or might not be the

Exhibit 1–4 Sample Lesson Plan

Short-term Objectives:

1. Steve will correctly produce the /s/ phoneme in all positions of words in 90% of his attempts.
2. Steve will correctly monitor (point to the appropriate light) his production of the /s/ phoneme in all positions in 90% of his attempts.
3. Steve will correctly imitate the /s/ phoneme in the initial position of words in sentences in 90% of his attempts.
4. Steve will correctly monitor (point to the appropriate light) his productions of the /s/ phoneme in the initial position of words in sentences in 90% of his attempts.
5. Steve will correctly produce the /s/ phoneme in the initial position of words in sentences in 90% of his attempts.
6. Steve will correctly monitor (point to the appropriate light) his productions of the /s/ phoneme in the initial position of words in sentences in 90% of his attempts.

Procedures:

1. Steve will say words containing the /s/ phoneme in the initial, medial, and final positions. If /s/ is produced incorrectly, auditory stimulation or placement cues will be used to help attain a correct response.
2. After saying each word, Steve will indicate the correctness of the /s/ production by pointing to a red light if incorrect and a green light if correct.
3. Sentences containing /s/ in the initial position of words will be presented for Steve to imitate. If errors are made, Steve will produce each errored word by itself. If correct production is attained, he will again imitate the sentence trying to incorporate this correct production. If production remains incorrect, the sentence will be broken into phrases and auditory stimulation will be used.
4. After imitating sentences containing /s/ in the initial position of words, Steve will indicate the correctness of each target production by pointing to a red light if incorrect and a green light if correct.
5. Steve will construct sentences containing /s/ in the initial position of words. If errors are made, he will produce each errored word by itself. If correct production is attained, Steve will again produce the sentence trying to incorporate this correct production.
6. After producing sentences containing the /s/ phoneme in the initial position of words, Steve will indicate the correctness of each target production by pointing to a red light if incorrect and a green light if correct.

---

same as terminal objectives that are the final objectives that need to be mastered prior to discharge. The length of time implied in "long-term" varies. It could mean 3 months or 1 year. "Long-term" has a built-in time frame, however, when one is functioning within a college or university setting. It has come to be defined as the length of one semester, one quarter, or two quarters depending on the administrative calendar. Thus, it seems reasonable that additional nomenclature could be "semester" or "quarter" objectives.

Objectives that can realistically be accomplished within the designated time frame must be determined. This task is not always easy and the initial long-range objectives may have to be revised at varying intervals. The number of revisions should decrease as experience is gained. Silverman (1984) stated, "Long-term goals specify the outcome the clinician is attempting to achieve" (p. 224). Because long-range objectives are written in a behavioral objective style, you should now have the foundation necessary for their construction.

The Relationship between Long-Range and Short-Range Objectives

Because short-range or short-term objectives are based on behavioral objectives, "short-term objectives must be consistent with the LTO [long-term objectives] and should flow from it" (Thompson 1977, p. 49). He also stated that short-range objectives "are small segments of behavior and should be manageable units of instruction [and] should assist the instructional process, not interfere with it" (pp. 50, 52). Thus it may be necessary for many short-range objectives to be accomplished before a long-range objective is achieved. For example, if a client cannot perform the following short-range objectives listed, it will be necessary to master them before being able to attain success on the long-term objective *(correct production of the /s/ phoneme in spontaneous conversation in 90% of his attempts)*. The client will:

1. auditorially discriminate (indicate by raising his hand) the /s/ phoneme from dissimilar phonemes when presented in isolation in 90% of his attempts,
2. auditorially discriminate (indicate by raising his hand) the /s/ phoneme from similar phonemes presented in isolation in 90% of his attempts,
3. auditorially discriminate (indicate by raising his hand) the /s/ phoneme from similar phonemes in consonant–vowel combinations in 90% of his attempts,
4. auditorially discriminate (indicate by raising his hand) the /s/ phoneme in the initial position of words when presented in rhyming word pairs in 90% of his attempts,
5. correctly imitate /s/ in isolation in 90% of his attempts,
6. correctly produce the /s/ phoneme in isolation in 90% of his attempts,
7. correctly monitor (state if correct or not) production of the /s/ phoneme in isolation in 90% of his attempts,

8. correctly imitate /s/ in the initial position of words in 90% of his attempts,
9. correctly produce /s/ in the initial position of words in 90% of his attempts,
10. correctly monitor (state if correct or not) production of the /s/ phoneme in the initial position of words in 90% of his attempts,
11. correctly produce /s/ in the final position of words in 90% of his attempts,
12. correctly monitor (state if correct or not) production of the /s/ phoneme in the final position of words in 90% of his attempts,
13. correctly produce /s/ in the initial position of words in phrases in 90% of his attempts,
14. correctly monitor (state if correct or not) production of the /s/ phoneme in the initial position of words in phrases in 90% of his attempts,
15. correctly produce /s/ in the initial and final positions of words in phrases in 90% of his attempts,
16. correctly monitor (state if correct or not) /s/ in the initial and final positions of words in phrases in 90% of his attempts,
17. correctly produce /s/ in the initial and final positions of words in sentences in 90% of his attempts,
18. correctly monitor (state if correct or not) /s/ in the initial and final positions of words in sentences in 90% of his attempts,
19. correctly produce /s/ in structured conversation in 90% of his attempts,
20. correctly monitor (self-correct) 90% of the incorrect /s/ productions during structured conversation.

Pending the client's progress, additional steps may have to be added, some may be combined, and some may be eliminated. For example, imitation of the target behavior may need to precede objectives 11, 13, 15, 17, and 19 if the client has difficulty with production. The client's performance will provide guidance in making these decisions. The point is that by accomplishing the listed short-range objectives, the client is working toward mastering the long-range objective. The end result is that if the client masters each short-range objective, he should be able to master the long-range objective, which is to correctly produce the /s/ phoneme in spontaneous conversation in 90% of his attempts.

A language example will be given to clarify further the relationship between long-range and short-range objectives. Again, it will be necessary for the client to master the short-range objectives that follow before being able to attain success on the long-range objective *(correct production of the singular present progressive tense in 90% of the obligatory contexts during all communication events)*. The client will:

1. correctly imitate Noun + is + Verb + ing immediately following a model in 90% of his attempts,
2. correctly imitate Noun + is + Verb + ing two seconds after the model is presented in 90% of his attempts,
3. correctly imitate Noun + is + Verb + ing when an intervening sentence is presented between the model and response in 90% of his attempts,
4. correctly produce Noun + is + Verb + ing in response to the question "What is the Noun doing?" in 90% of his attempts,
5. correctly produce Noun + is + Verb + ing in response to "What's happening in this picture?" in 90% of his attempts,
6. correctly produce Noun + is + Verb + ing in response to "Tell me about the Noun" in 90% of the obligatory contexts,
7. correctly produce Noun + is + Verb + ing when telling a story from pictures in 90% of the obligatory contexts,
8. correctly produce Noun + is + Verb + ing when looking out the window and discussing events of the people seen in 90% of the obligatory contexts,
9. correctly produce Noun + is + Verb + ing during an oral presentation in the classroom in 90% of all obligatory contexts.

The client's performance determines when and whether other steps should be added, combined, or eliminated. By accomplishing the short-range objectives just listed, the client is working toward mastery of the long-range objective. If the client successfully passes through the various steps, he is well on his way toward correct production of the singular present progressive tense in obligatory contexts encountered during communication events.

Relationship between Long-Range and Terminal Objectives

It was previously mentioned that long-range objectives might or might not be the same as the terminal objectives that are also based on behavioral objectives. An explanation that focuses on the two long-range objectives discussed in the previous section is provided in this section. The articulation objective is *correct production of the /s/ phoneme in spontaneous conversation in 90% of his attempts*. The language objective is *correct production of the singular present progressive tense in 90% of the obligatory contexts during all communication events*.

If a client with an articulation problem only misarticulates the /s/ phoneme and has no other speech, language, or communication problem, the long-range objective just stated is the same as the terminal objective, which Mowrer (1988) says is "one you wish to have accomplished when you are ready to dismiss a case"

(p. 169). In other words, as soon as the client masters the long-range objective, he will be discharged or terminated from therapy. If the client misarticulates other phonemes that he should have mastered, therapy will continue. In this latter example, the long-range objective and terminal objective are not synonymous. The client's terminal objective may be *correct production of the /s/, /l/, and /r/ phonemes in all contexts during spontaneous conversation in 90% of his attempts.* The objective can also be stated as *correct production of all phonemes in all contexts during spontaneous conversation in 90% of his attempts.*

Likewise, the long-range language objective can be a terminal objective under certain circumstances. If the rest of the client's language, speech, and communication is appropriate for his age, he will be dismissed from therapy when the present progressive tense is mastered. Thus, this long-range objective is the same as a terminal objective in this situation. If, however, the client has difficulty with other aspects of language, other long-range objectives have to be mastered before being discharged from therapy. In this latter case, a long-range objective and a terminal objective differ.

If the client will be dismissed from therapy upon attainment of an objective, it can be considered a terminal objective. If the client will be returning for additional therapy, an objective is not terminal.

Reports

Behavioral objectives are found in both the initial evaluation and the progress report. Because these reports are usually required at the end of the semester or quarter, they are sometimes called "end of the semester progress reports" or "quarter progress reports." The objectives that will be emphasized in therapy are listed in the initial evaluation. These objectives are again included in the end of the semester or quarter progress report, followed by an account of the actual progress made during the designated time frame. These reports are discussed in a later chapter but are mentioned here because it is important to understand the extent to which behavioral objectives are used in the speech-language pathology profession.

Individualized Education Plan

The term *individualized education plan* (IEP), which had its origin in The Education for All Handicapped Children Act of 1975 (P.L. 94-142), is very familiar to those working in the field of education. According to P.L. 94-142, an IEP is a written statement for a handicapped child that describes the educational objectives for that child and the special services to be provided. The IEP process will become increasingly important and take on more significance when fulfilling student teaching requirements in a public school setting. In the school setting, the term *IEP,* is more widely used than is behavioral or instructional objective. The law requires that IEPs include annual goals and short-term instructional objectives. Thus, knowledge of behavioral objectives is incorporated into IEP writing.

CONCLUSION

A goal that you should accomplish as early as possible in the clinical practicum process is to understand the composition and construction of well-written behavioral objectives. Behavioral objectives have far-reaching effects, as they form the basis for much of the paperwork required in speech-language pathology. Being able to write behavioral objectives skillfully and realize their importance during this part of the clinical experience can only enhance future professional performance.

KNOW IT! USE IT!

After reading this chapter, you should be able to:

1. state three reasons why behavioral objectives are important
2. state and explain the three components of a behavioral objective
3. divide behavioral objectives into components in 90% of your attempts
4. correctly write behavioral objectives in 90% of your attempts

---

REFERENCES

The Education for All Handicapped Children Act of 1975, Pub. L. No. 94-142.

Mager, R.F. (1984). *Preparing instructional objectives* (rev. 2nd ed.). Belmont, CA: Fearon.

Mowrer, D.E. (1988). *Methods of modifying speech behaviors* (2nd ed.). Prospect Heights, IL: Waveland Press.

Silverman, F.H. (1984). *Speech-language pathology and audiology: An introduction.* Columbus, OH: Merrill.

Thompson, D.G. (1977). *Writing long-term and short-term objectives.* Campaign: Research Press.

Wheeler, A.H., & Fox, W.L. (1977). *A guide to writing instructional objectives.* Lawrence, KS: H&H Enterprises.

Identifying Components of Behavioral Objectives— Exercise

The lead-in, *The client will . . .,* is used for all examples in this section. Read the following sample objectives and figure out the *performance, condition,* and *criterion* for each. Write these aspects on the lines provided. When completed, check your responses with Appendix 1–B.

Sample Objectives 1: Articulation

1. correctly produce the /r/ phoneme in all positions of words in 90% of his attempts
    * Performance: _____
    * Condition: _____
    * Criterion: _____
2. correctly imitate /s/ in isolation in 8 of 10 attempts
    * Performance: _____
    * Condition: _____
    * Criterion: _____
3. raise his tongue tip to the alveolar ridge with his mouth opened at least 1½ inches on 8 of 10 trials
    * Performance: _____
    * Condition: _____
    * Criterion: _____
4. auditorially discriminate (by raising his hand) /s/ from /f/ in consonant-vowel combinations in 90% of his attempts.
    * Performance: _____
    * Condition: _____
    * Criterion: _____
5. correctly monitor (state if correct or not) production of the /l/ phoneme during spontaneous conversation in 90% of his attempts
    * Performance: _____

- Condition: _____
- Criterion: _____

6. correctly monitor (self-correct) 90% of the incorrect /s/ productions during reading
   - Performance: _____
   - Condition: _____
   - Criterion: _____

Sample Objectives 2: Phonology

1. close syllables on spontaneously produced monosyllabic target words in 90% of his attempts (Note: This objective addresses the process deletion of final consonants.)
   - Performance: _____
   - Condition: _____
   - Criterion: _____

2. correctly imitate the consonant clusters /sk/, /sp/, and /st/ without a pause between the two consonants in 90% of his attempts (Note: This objective addresses the process cluster reduction.)
   - Performance: _____
   - Condition: _____
   - Criterion: _____

3. produce unstressed syllables in bisyllabic words in 90% of his attempts (Note: This objective addresses the process deletion of unstressed syllables.)
   - Performance: _____
   - Condition: _____
   - Criterion: _____

4. produce voiceless consonants when preceding vowels in 90% of the appropriate contexts (Note: This objective addresses the process prevocalic voicing of consonants.)
   - Performance: _____
   - Condition: _____
   - Criterion: _____

5. produce fricatives or affricates in 90% of the appropriate contexts (Note: This objective addresses the process stopping.)
   - Performance: _____
   - Condition: _____
   - Criterion: _____

6. produce liquids in 90% of the appropriate contexts (Note: This objective addresses the process gliding.)
   * Performance: _____
   * Condition: _____
   * Criterion: _____

Sample Objectives 3: Language

1. spontaneously name 20 of 25 pictures in a children's dictionary
   * Performance: _____
   * Condition: _____
   * Criterion: _____

2. expressively identify (name) pictures of common objects in 90% of his attempts
   * Performance: _____
   * Condition: _____
   * Criterion: _____

3. receptively identify (point to) pictures given in a field of three in 8 of 10 attempts
   * Performance: _____
   * Condition: _____
   * Criterion: _____

4. correctly use present progressive tense while describing 20 of 25 pictures that are not visible to the clinician
   * Performance: _____
   * Condition: _____
   * Criterion: _____

5. appropriately use the pronouns "he" and "she" during conversation in 90% of his attempts
   * Performance: _____
   * Condition: _____
   * Criterion: _____

6. correctly use regular plurals in at least 90% of his attempts while telling a story
   * Performance: _____
   * Condition: _____
   * Criterion: _____

Sample Objectives 4: Voice

1. identify (by raising his hand) at least seven of his vocal abuses when all possible abuses are stated
   - Performance: _____
   - Condition: _____
   - Criterion: _____
2. explain three steps in laryngeal functioning one session after the clinician's explanation
   - Performance: _____
   - Condition: _____
   - Criterion: _____
3. use appropriate pitch while producing /ɑ/ in 8 of 10 trials
   - Performance: _____
   - Condition: _____
   - Criterion: _____
4. produce easy onset of voice on the vowels /o/ and /i/ in 90% of his attempts
   - Performance: _____
   - Condition: _____
   - Criterion: _____
5. produce appropriate oral resonance on vowel–consonant combinations in 90% of his attempts
   - Performance: _____
   - Condition: _____
   - Criterion: _____

Sample Objectives 5: Fluency

1. identify (by saying "there") 90% of his nonfluencies that consist of prolongations lasting longer than 2 seconds
   - Performance: _____
   - Condition: _____
   - Criterion: _____
2. read in front of his class with less than 0.5 stuttered words per minute
   - Performance: _____
   - Condition: _____
   - Criterion: _____
3. speak with less than 0.5 stuttered words per minute during 5 minutes of spontaneous conversation with the clinician
   - Performance: _____

- Condition: _____
- Criterion: _____

4. cancel 90% of the stuttering episodes that occur while talking on the telephone
   - Performance: _____
   - Condition: _____
   - Criterion: _____

5. identify (state) all factors in his stuttering equation one session after this discussion occurred
   - Performance: _____
   - Condition: _____
   - Criterion: _____

6. use pull-outs during all episodes of blocking while speaking to the principal for 5 minutes
   - Performance: _____
   - Condition: _____
   - Criterion: _____

Sample Objectives 6: Pragmatics

1. request (by pointing or using eye gaze) an object that is out of reach twice during a 10-minute time segment
   - Performance: _____
   - Condition: _____
   - Criterion: _____

2. take three consecutive turns when a familiar joint action routine is initiated by a significant other
   - Performance: _____
   - Condition: _____
   - Criterion: _____

3. attend to (look at) the speaker during two of three communication episodes
   - Performance: _____
   - Condition: _____
   - Criterion: _____

4. initiate a greeting upon seeing the clinician on four of five appropriate occasions
   - Performance: _____
   - Condition: _____
   - Criterion: _____

5. specify a topic once during each therapy session
   - Performance: _____
   - Condition: _____
   - Criterion: _____
6. maintain a topic initiated by someone else for three conversational turns
   - Performance: _____
   - Condition: _____
   - Criterion: _____

Sample Objectives 7: Problem Behavior
1. walk into the therapy room without yanking the clinician's arm in two of the three weekly therapy sessions
   - Performance: _____
   - Condition: _____
   - Criterion: _____
2. sit without kicking for 5 minutes after the removal of restraints [your hands on the client's knees]
   - Performance: _____
   - Condition: _____
   - Criterion: _____
3. attend to (look at) a picture for 2 minutes when a desirable toy is within reaching distance
   - Performance: _____
   - Condition: _____
   - Criterion: _____
4. perform a specified task for 25 minutes without throwing a temper tantrum
   - Performance: _____
   - Condition: _____
   - Criterion: _____
5. follow 8 of 10 directions within 2 seconds of the initial presentation
   - Performance: _____
   - Condition: _____
   - Criterion: _____

Identifying Components of Behavioral Objectives— Answers

Sample Objectives 1: Articulation

1. correctly produce the /r/ phoneme in all positions of words in 90% of his attempts
   - Performance: *correctly produce the /r/ phoneme*
   - Condition: *in all positions of words*
   - Criterion: *in 90% of his attempts*
2. correctly imitate /s/ in isolation in 8 of 10 attempts
   - Performance: *correctly imitate /s/*
   - Condition: *in isolation*
   - Criterion: *in 8 of 10 attempts*
3. raise his tongue tip to the alveolar ridge with his mouth opened at least 1½ inches on 8 of 10 trials
   - Performance: *raise his tongue tip to the alveolar ridge*
   - Condition: *with his mouth opened at least 1½ inches*
   - Criterion: *on 8 of 10 trials*
4. auditorially discriminate (by raising his hand) /s/ from /f/ in consonant-vowel combinations in 90% of his attempts
   - Performance: *auditorially discriminate (by raising his hand) /s/ from /f/*
   - Condition: *in consonant–vowel combinations*
   - Criterion: *in 90% of his attempts*
5. correctly monitor (state if correct or not) production of the /l/ phoneme during spontaneous conversation in 90% of his attempts
   - Performance: *correctly monitor (state if correct or not) production of the /l/ phoneme*

- Condition: *during spontaneous conversation*
- Criterion: *in 90% of his attempts*

6. correctly monitor (self-correct) 90% of the incorrect /s/ productions during reading
   - Performance: *correctly monitor (self-correct) incorrect /s/ productions*
   - Condition: *during reading*
   - Criterion: *90%*

Sample Objectives 2: Phonology

1. close syllables on spontaneously produced monosyllabic target words in 90% of his attempts (Note: This objective addresses the process deletion of final consonants.)
   - Performance: *close syllables*
   - Condition: *on spontaneously produced monosyllabic target words*
   - Criterion: *in 90% of his attempts*

2. correctly imitate the consonant clusters /sk/, /sp/, and /st/ without a pause between the two consonants in 90% of his attempts (Note: This objective addresses the process cluster reduction.)
   - Performance: *correctly imitate the consonant clusters /sk/, /sp/, and /st/*
   - Condition: *without a pause between the two consonants*
   - Criterion: *in 90% of his attempts*

3. produce unstressed syllables in bisyllabic words in 90% of his attempts (Note: This objective addresses the process deletion of unstressed syllables.)
   - Performance: *produce unstressed syllables*
   - Condition: *in bisyllabic words*
   - Criterion: *in 90% of his attempts*

4. produce voiceless consonants when preceding vowels in 90% of the appropriate contexts (Note: This objective addresses the process prevocalic voicing of consonants.)
   - Performance: *produce voiceless consonants*
   - Condition: *when preceding vowels*
   - Criterion: *in 90% of the appropriate contexts*

5. produce fricatives or affricates in 90% of the appropriate contexts (Note: This objective addresses the process stopping.)
   - Performance: *produce fricatives or affricates*
   - Condition: *the appropriate contexts*
   - Criterion: *90%*

6. produce liquids in 90% of the appropriate contexts (Note: This objective addresses the process gliding.)
   - Performance: produce liquids
   - Condition: the appropriate contexts
   - Criterion: 90%

Sample Objectives 3: Language

1. spontaneously name 20 of 25 pictures in a children's dictionary
   - Performance: spontaneously name pictures
   - Condition: in a children's dictionary
   - Criterion: 20 of 25
2. expressively identify (name) pictures of common objects in 90% of his attempts
   - Performance: expressively identify (name) pictures
   - Condition: of common objects
   - Criterion: in 90% of his attempts
3. receptively identify (point to) pictures given in a field of three in 8 of 10 attempts
   - Performance: receptively identify (point to) pictures
   - Condition: given in a field of three
   - Criterion: in 8 of 10 attempts
4. correctly use present progressive tense while describing 20 of 25 pictures that are not visible to the clinician
   - Performance: correctly use present progressive tense
   - Condition: while describing pictures that are not visible to the clinician
   - Criterion: 20 of 25
5. appropriately use the pronouns "he" and "she" during conversation in 90% of his attempts
   - Performance: appropriately use the pronouns "he" and "she"
   - Condition: during conversation
   - Criterion: in 90% of his attempts
6. correctly use regular plurals in at least 90% of his attempts while telling a story
   - Performance: correctly use regular plurals
   - Condition: while telling a story
   - Criterion: in at least 90% of his attempts

Sample Objectives 4: Voice

1. identify (by raising his hand) at least seven of his vocal abuses when all possible abuses are stated

- Performance: identify (by raising his hand) vocal abuses
- Condition: when all possible abuses are stated
- Criterion: at least seven

2. explain three steps in laryngeal functioning one session after the clinician's explanation
   - Performance: explain steps in laryngeal functioning
   - Condition: one session after the clinician's explanation
   - Criterion: three

3. use appropriate pitch while producing /ɑ/ in 8 of 10 trials
   - Performance: use appropriate pitch
   - Condition: while producing /ɑ/
   - Criterion: in 8 of 10 trials

4. produce easy onset of voice on the vowels /o/ and /i/ in 90% of his attempts
   - Performance: produce easy onset of voice
   - Condition: on the vowels /o/ and /i/
   - Criterion: in 90% of his attempts

5. produce appropriate oral resonance on vowel–consonant combinations in 90% of his attempts.
   - Performance: produce appropriate oral resonance
   - Condition: on vowel–consonant combinations
   - Criterion: in 90% of his attempts

Sample Objectives 5: Fluency

1. identify (by saying "there") 90% of his nonfluencies that consist of prolongations lasting longer than 2 seconds
   - Performance: identify (by saying "there") his nonfluencies
   - Condition: that consist of prolongations lasting longer than 2 seconds
   - Criterion: 90% of his nonfluencies

2. read in front of his class with less than 0.5 stuttered words per minute
   - Performance: read
   - Condition: in front of his class
   - Criterion: with less than 0.5 stuttered words per minute

3. speak with less than 0.5 stuttered words per minute during 5 minutes of spontaneous conversation with the clinician
   - Performance: speak
   - Condition: during 5 minutes of spontaneous conversation with the clinician
   - Criterion: with less than 0.5 stuttered words per minute

4. cancel 90% of the stuttering episodes that occur while talking on the telephone
   - Performance: *cancel stuttering episodes*
   - Condition: *that occur while talking on the telephone*
   - Criterion: *90%*

5. identify (state) all factors in his stuttering equation one session after this discussion occurred
   - Performance: *identify (state) factors in his stuttering equation*
   - Condition: *one session after this discussion occurred*
   - Criterion: *all*

6. use pull-outs during all episodes of blocking while speaking to the principal for 5 minutes.
   - Performance: *use pull-outs during episodes of blocking*
   - Condition: *while speaking to the principal for 5 minutes*
   - Criterion: *all*

Sample Objectives 6: Pragmatics

1. request (by pointing or using eye gaze) an object that is out of reach twice during a 10-minute time segment
   - Performance: *request (by pointing or using eye gaze) an object*
   - Condition: *that is out of reach*
   - Criterion: *twice during a 10-minute time segment*

2. take three consecutive turns when a familiar joint action routine is initiated by a significant other
   - Performance: *take consecutive turns*
   - Condition: *when a familiar joint action routine is initiated by a significant other*
   - Criterion: *three*

3. attend to (look at) the speaker during two of three communication episodes
   - Performance: *attend to (look at) the speaker*
   - Condition: *during communication episodes*
   - Criterion: *two of three*

4. initiate a greeting upon seeing the clinician on four of five appropriate occasions
   - Performance: *initiate a greeting*
   - Condition: *upon seeing the clinician*
   - Criterion: *on four of five appropriate occasions*

5. specify a topic once during each therapy session
   - Performance: specify a topic
   - Condition: during each therapy session
   - Criterion: once
6. maintain a topic initiated by someone else for three conversational turns
   - Performance: maintain a topic
   - Condition: initiated by someone else
   - Criterion: for three conversational turns

Sample Objectives 7: Problem Behavior

1. walk into the therapy room without yanking the clinician's arm in two of the three weekly therapy sessions
   - Performance: walk into the therapy room
   - Condition: without yanking the clinician's arm
   - Criterion: in two of the three weekly therapy sessions
2. sit without kicking for 5 minutes after the removal of restraints [your hands on the client's knees]
   - Performance: sit without ki cking
   - Condition: after the removal of restraints
   - Criterion: for 5 minutes
3. attend to (look at) a picture for 2 minutes when a desirable toy is within reaching distance
   - Performance: attend to (look at) a picture
   - Condition: when a desirable toy is within reaching distance
   - Criterion: for 2 minutes
4. perform a specified task for 25 minutes without throwing a temper tantrum
   - Performance: perform a specified task
   - Condition: without throwing a temper tantrum
   - Criterion: for 25 minutes
5. follow 8 of 10 directions within 2 seconds of the initial presentation
   - Performance: follow directions
   - Condition: within 2 seconds of the initial presentation
   - Criterion: 8 of 10

If you correctly identified at least 90% of the components in this exercise and are satisfied with your performance, return to where you left off in chapter 1 and begin reading the section entitled *Application and Importance of Behavioral Objectives*.

CHAPTER 2

Behavioral Objectives: Common Writing Problems

CHAPTER HIGHLIGHTS

- *problems to avoid while writing behavioral objectives*
- *writing problem-free behavioral objectives*
- *critically analyzing behavioral objectives*

After many semesters of reading and discussing behavioral objectives with students in the three stages of clinical training, it becomes apparent to supervisors that more background information must be provided to students so they can write behavioral objectives in a clear and acceptable fashion. When you are in the new status of "beginning clinician," you do not always know why behavioral objectives just cannot include performance, condition, and criterion components. Why, you might wonder, must behavioral objectives be written in a particular manner? When your objectives are not approved, you do not always understand how to improve them. In this chapter, common problems in *writing* behavioral objectives will be discussed to clarify how to prepare well-written objectives in speech-language pathology.

OBJECTIVES PROBLEM 1: INCORRECT FORMAT FOLLOWING THE LEAD-IN

Problems with the portion of the objective immediately following the "lead-in," or introductory statement, occur frequently. This is easy to correct because it involves a lack of consistency between the lead-in and the actual objective. The "lead-in" is the introductory statement that precedes the list of behavioral objectives and is followed by a colon. However, the problem results from not following all rules specific to the colon's usage. If the portion following the colon is a complete sentence, it should begin with an uppercase letter. If the portion following the colon is not a complete sentence, it should begin with a lower case letter. To demonstrate, examples from beginning clinicians will be given. Beginning clinician examples will be coded with a "U" (for *uncorrected*) following the number. These examples are highlighted and set in boldface. Corrected versions will be coded with "C" (for *corrected*) following the corresponding number of the clinician. The new or corrected information is underlined.

The first example, as it appeared on a beginning clinician's lesson plan, follows. To avoid confusion when reading the example, "Lesson objectives:" was the lead-in used, which will be assumed throughout this chapter.

1.1(U) the client will receptively identify (by pointing) 8 of 10 body parts.

Because the portion following the colon is a complete sentence, "the" should begin with an uppercase letter. A correct way to state this objective is:

1.1(C) <u>The</u> client will receptively identify (by pointing) 8 of 10 body parts.

QUICK CHECK

The "lead-in" is the introductory statement that precedes the list of behavioral objectives and is followed by a colon. If the portion following the colon is a complete sentence, the first word should be capitalized. If the portion following the colon is not a complete sentence, the first word should begin with a lowercase letter.

OBJECTIVES PROBLEM 2: CONSISTENCY

Another problem frequently occurs when more than one objective is cited. It deals with the lack of consistency with which the objectives are written. An example is:

2.1(U) Scott will spontaneously produce two-word combinations twice during the session.

to correctly imitate Noun + Verb + Object combinations presented while looking at a storybook in 90% of his attempts

This example clearly shows a lack of consistency in the structure of the objectives. All objectives cited together should begin in the same manner. Either of the formats shown can be used. Examples of each type follow:

2.1(C.1) **<u>to</u> spontaneously produce two-word combinations twice during the session**

<u>to</u> correctly imitate Noun + Verb + Object combinations presented while looking at a storybook in 90% of his attempts

or

2.1(C.2) **<u>Scott</u> will spontaneously produce two-word combinations twice during the session.**

<u>Scott</u> will correctly imitate Noun + Verb + Object combinations presented while looking at a storybook in 90% of his attempts.

> **QUICK CHECK**
>
> It is important to be consistent when writing objectives. Adopt one format and stick with it!

OBJECTIVES PROBLEM 3: PERFORMANCE COMPONENT

One problem encountered in the performance component is the use of verbs that are not specific. This aspect was discussed at length in chapter 1. An example of an objective containing this error is:

3.1(U) **to discriminate among the /s/ phoneme and other phonemes in 7 of 10 attempts**

The verb *discriminate* is not directly observable. Thus, an indicator behavior is needed. If it is not present, it is not possible to know exactly what the client will be doing when demonstrating achievement of the objective. An example of this correction is as follows:

3.1(C.1) **to discriminate <u>auditorially</u> (by raising his hand) among the /s/ phoneme and other phonemes in 7 of 10 attempts**

The indicator behavior ("by raising his hand") takes care of the initial problem. However, one must remember that anyone reading the objective should be able *to picture* the task to be performed. If "auditorially" is not included, one can conceivably expect a visual task in which the client raises his hand when shown the letter "S" and does not raise it when another letter is shown. If, however, one knows the definition of a phoneme, this interpretation is excluded, but another exists. A deaf child may be discriminating the /s/ phoneme from other phonemes solely through the visual modality—how each phoneme looks when produced. These possibilities are included to stress the importance of critically reading and evaluating objectives. The development of these skills should result in better written objectives.

To narrow the focus further, this objective could be still more specific. From the original objective, it is questionable if this beginning clinician really knew where she was headed in the remediation process. Further information on the nature of "other phonemes" should be provided. Is the client being required to make gross or fine discriminations? This information can be provided in more than one way. Two suggestions are:

3.1(C.2) to discriminate auditorially (by raising his hand) the /s/ phoneme <u>from all other fricatives</u> in 70% of his attempts

or

3.1(C.3) to discriminate auditorially (by raising his hand) the /s/ phoneme from /f, v, θ, ð, z, ʃ/, and /ʒ/ presented in isolation in 70% of his attempts

This objective is now well written. Problems with the performance aspect have been rectified and a condition has been added to eliminate ambiguity.

An example of a second problem occurring in the performance component follows. This problem may not be obvious on initial scrutiny, but it should become apparent.

3.2(U) to discuss with Larry the visual and acoustic characteristics of the /s/ phoneme

Please keep in mind that the performance component is being discussed. Problems dealing with the other components will be corrected in the objective but not discussed in this section. The major problem with the performance part of the objective is that the focus is misplaced. It is on the wrong person. The performance aspect is supposed to deal with what the learner or client does while demonstrating achievement of an objective and not what you, the clinician, does. The following revision in the performance component places the emphasis on the client. It is:

3.2(C) to state two visual and two acoustic characteristics of the /s/ phoneme

This objective clearly states what the client has to do to be successful. Another objective is as follows:

3.3(U) to produce the /s/ phoneme in words with 90% accuracy

Here the problem in the performance component may not be initially obvious. The client may already be producing an /s/ phoneme, but it may be distorted. According to the manner in which this objective is written, distorted /s/ productions would be considered correct. This revised objective does not consider distortions acceptable. It is:

3.3(C) to produce the /s/ phoneme correctly in all positions of words in 90% of his attempts

The impact of simply adding *correctly* is important. This change is not insignificant when its implications are understood.

The next example states what the client will do, but the manner in which it is stated is not clear and precise:

3.4(U) to produce the /s/ phoneme in sentences by imitation with 90% accuracy.

The word *imitation* is a key word in the objective, as it states exactly what the client will be doing. Thus, it should receive more emphasis. A revised objective is:

3.4(C) to imitate the /s/ phoneme correctly in sentences in 90% of his attempts

Note that the word *imitate* is more strategically placed. Therefore, it will be less likely to be overlooked. The inaccurate impression from reading objective 3.4(U) is that the client is spontaneously producing the phoneme in sentences. This conclusion is not reflected in the revised objective 3.4(C). Behavioral objectives must be written in a precise and specific manner so that misinterpretation does not result.

When looking at the next objective, continue to keep in mind what the client should be doing while demonstrating achievement. If this aspect cannot be determined from the objective, it is not well written. For example,

3.5(U) to strengthen and stabilize the /s/ phoneme in 90% of her attempts

The words *strengthen* and *stabilize* are recognized as being a part of Van Riper and Emerick's (1990) articulation therapy program, but they are not used precisely enough here to know exactly what the client will be doing. Many therapeutic techniques will lead to strengthening and stabilization of a particular phoneme if executed skillfully. Therefore, the performance component must be more specific. Two possible corrections are:

3.5(C.1)   to prolong correct production of the /s/ phoneme in isolation for 15 seconds

and/or

3.5(C.2)   to produce the /s/ phoneme correctly in isolation 15 times in 15 seconds

Both of these objectives provide a clear idea of what the client must do in order to demonstrate achievement.

In this section, problems affecting the performance component of behavioral objectives have been identified and discussed. Example one showed usage of a nonspecific verb. It also showed that the entire objective had to be written in a more specific manner. Example two placed the focus on the clinician instead of on the client. By not clearly stating the intention in the third example, distorted productions were acceptable. In other words, the actual intent did not come across to others reading the objective. Example four conveyed the idea that the objective should be broken down into the smallest, most precise behavior and should clearly reflect what the client was supposed to do. Example five does not specifically state what the client should do.

QUICK CHECK

There are a few important points to remember when constructing the performance portion of a behavioral objective. Be certain it reflects exactly what the client will do in order to demonstrate achievement of the objective. Be certain that the verbs used are specific.

OBJECTIVES PROBLEM 4: CONDITION COMPONENT

Problems encountered in this component stem from either not stating or not clearly stating the circumstances under, or in, which the performance is done. Problems concerning components other than the condition are corrected in these revisions but are not discussed in this section. The first example is:

4.1(U) to determine the location of the /t/ phoneme with 90% accuracy

The reader cannot readily determine the nature of this task. Thus, more description is necessary. An acceptable revision is: .

4.1(C) to determine (by pointing to train cars) the correct location of the /t/ phoneme <u>when three phonemes are presented in isolation</u> in 90% of his attempts

This revised objective enables the reader to predetermine the task that will be presented. The initial objective 4.1(U) did not specify the environment in which the /t/ phoneme would be presented. Specifically, would the /t/ phoneme be presented in isolation, syllables, words, or sentences? In the revised objective, there is no guesswork involved, as the unit (isolation) is clearly specified in the condition aspect of the objective.

This next example further illustrates how the condition in an objective adds clarification. This objective is:

4.2(U) to discriminate auditorially between the /p/ and /b/ phonemes in 90% of her attempts

To avoid misinterpretation, further clarification is necessary. This aspect is accomplished by including a condition in the objective. A revised objective is:

4.2(C) to discriminate correctly and auditorially (<u>by pointing to the corresponding picture</u>) between the /p/ and /b/ phonemes <u>presented in isolation</u> in 90% of her attempts (Note: A picture of a motor boat is associated with /p/ and a picture of a ball is associated with /b/ on this particular task.)

The conditions *by pointing to the corresponding picture* and *presented in isolation* clarify the task. The reader is now given enough information to develop a preconceived notion about the therapeutic task that the clinician and client will be performing to accomplish the objective. A well-defined objective is also likely to keep the clinician on task.

The next example gives an impression of a client functioning on a higher level than he actually is.

4.3(U) to produce the /s/ phoneme correctly in sentences in 54 of 60 attempts

When reading this objective, the idea that the client can spontaneously produce sentences and maintain correct /s/ production is conveyed; however, the client is not performing at this level. Thus, a condition needs to be stated in the objective.

4.3(C) to produce the /s/ words correctly <u>on his word list when incorporated into sentences</u> in 90% of his attempts

The fact that the client's production centered around incorporating a word containing the /s/ phoneme into a sentence indicates that a reminder is necessary in order for correct production to be achieved. When the objective is worded in this manner, one gets a more realistic idea of the level at which the client is functioning.

Notice how much more specific the next objective becomes when a condition is added.

4.4(U) to produce the /p/, /t/, /k/, and /v/ phonemes correctly in syllables in four of five attempts

As written, the objective indicates that the client will be producing all syllable types. If one thinks of all the different possibilities, it makes sense to add a clarifying statement or condition. This addition is reflected in the revision.

4.4(C) to produce each of these phonemes /p, t, k/, and /v/ correctly in <u>consonant–vowel combinations</u> in four of five attempts

The condition *consonant–vowel combinations* limits the type of syllable that will be produced.

In the next example, the condition also needs clarification.

4.5(U) to receptively identify 13 of 15 objects correctly

The impression obtained from reading this objective is that 15 objects will be placed in front of the client. He will be responsible for selecting the object named from the entire field of 15. This is not, however, the intent. Thus the goal needs to be revised. It is:

4.5(C) to receptively identify <u>(point to)</u> 13 of 15 objects <u>correctly given a field of two</u>

This objective as written indicates that two objects will be presented to the client at a time. Selecting one object from a field of 15 is a much more difficult task than selecting an object from a field of two. When the objective is worded in this manner, it is less likely to be misinterpreted.

Objectives containing problems in the condition component have been discussed. In all examples, the revisions consist of adding additional information that describes the circumstances under, or in, which the performance is to be done.

QUICK CHECK

Important information to keep in mind with regard to the condition component is to be as specific as possible. Include pertinent and relevant situations and circumstances in the objective that are necessary for clarification so that misinterpretation is prevented.

OBJECTIVES PROBLEM 5: CRITERION COMPONENT

This component deals with how well the client is expected to perform. Problems encountered in this area arise from either not stating a criterion or not stating it accurately. The first example lacks a criterion.

5.1(U) to produce the /s/ phoneme correctly in isolation

Because a criterion is not stated, it is not possible to know when the objective has been accomplished. A revision is as follows:

5.1(C) to produce the /s/ phoneme correctly in isolation <u>in 90% of his attempts</u>

It is now possible to know when the objective is accomplished as well as measure the client's progress.

Technically, there is nothing wrong with the manner in which the criterion is stated in this second objective. It is, however, needlessly binding.

5.2(U) to produce the /s/ phoneme correctly in sentences in 54 of 60 attempts

Strictly speaking, there is no way the client can meet this criterion if he is not given 60 tries to produce /s/. If the child produces 40 sentences (each containing one /s/ phoneme) and correctly produces 36 of the /s/ phonemes, he cannot meet the criterion despite the high level of success (90%). Further, by stating the criterion in this manner, flexibility is stifled because it is not possible to move to another objective until the client has been given 60 opportunities to produce /s/. If the objective was written differently, this would not happen. For example:

5.2(C) to produce the /s/ phoneme correctly in sentences <u>in 90% of his attempts</u>

Stating the objective in this manner *is* conducive to flexibility. Moving to a higher level objective is contingent on the client's performance alone and not on an arbitrary number of trials. More specifically, if the client correctly produces 9 of 10 /s/ phonemes, he has met the criterion and can move to a higher level objective. Additional time does not have to be spent getting 50 more trials. The percentage of success is 90% for both objectives, but the second way is clearly less restrictive and permits more effective use of time and allows more efficient and flexible therapy.

The next example is more abstract. The term *accuracy,* here defined as *correctness,* leads to confusion in this objective.

5.3(U) to produce the /s/ phoneme in isolation with 90% accuracy in all attempts

This objective can be paraphrased by saying that every time the client produces the /s/ phoneme, his production will be 90% accurate. This can be interpreted as meaning that the /s/ phoneme will not be totally correct because this would be indicated by 100% accurate. Ninety percent accuracy implies that the production is not quite right. Would this be equivalent to a distorted /s/ production? The revised objective is not as prone to multiple interpretations. It is:

5.3(C) to produce the /s/ phoneme correctly in isolation <u>in 90% of her attempts</u>

This criterion clearly indicates that the client must produce the /s/ phoneme correctly in at least 90% of the total number of attempts. If the total number of trials is 50, the client has to produce /s/ correctly in at least 45 of them in order to meet criterion.

This next objective is written in a sloppy and imprecise manner. The meaning is nearly beyond comprehension.

5.4(U) to produce the /s/ target phoneme in isolation 30 times in 100% of her attempts

This reader interprets this objective as meaning that the client will produce the /s/ phoneme 30 times and that it has to be correct each time in order to meet criterion. To write this objective in a less confusing manner, it is suggested that one determines what is important. Is it the number 30 or 100% of the attempts or both? If both are important, the objective can be revised as follows:

5.4(C.1) to produce the /s/ phoneme correctly in isolation <u>in 30 of 30 attempts</u>

or

5.4(C.2) to produce the /s/ phoneme correctly in isolation <u>in all 30 attempts</u>

Another issue arises. A criterion of 90% is adequate because it is expected that a client will continue to improve after training stops. It is not efficient to work on a behavior that will continue to show some spontaneous improvement. Thus, it is suggested that the original objective be revised from "100% of her attempts" to 90% to allow for spontaneous growth. The revised objective is:

5.4(C.3) to produce the /s/ phoneme correctly in isolation <u>in 90% of her attempts</u>

If it is decided that the number 30 is important, the objective can be written in a couple of ways. One is:

5.4(C.4) to produce the /s/ phoneme correctly in isolation <u>in 30 consecutive trials</u>

If the trials do not have to be consecutive, the objective can be stated in this manner:

5.4(C.5) to produce the /s/ phoneme correctly in isolation <u>a total of 30 times</u>

Stated this latter way, the number of trials is not important. The client can meet the criterion by producing /s/ in isolation correctly in 30 of 60 trials or in 30 of 70 trials. Stating the criterion in this manner is not suggested, as the client can meet it without having adequate success and without actual mastery of the phoneme. For example, in the former example, the client's percentage of correctness is 50%. In the latter example, it is 43%. Neither of these percentages warrants progressing to a higher level objective.

This next objective does not state the criterion clearly.

5.5(U) to produce the target /s/ phoneme in isolation in 90% of his attempts 25 times

After discussing the other four objectives in this section, you will probably be able to revise this objective immediately. Two suggested revisions are:

5.5(C.1) to produce the /s/ phoneme correctly in isolation <u>in 90% of his attempts</u>

or

5.5(C.2) to produce the /s/ phoneme correctly in isolation <u>in 23 of 25 attempts</u>

The first revision is more acceptable than the second because it enables more flexibility. (This aspect was presented during discussion of the second objective in this section.)

Problems specific to the criterion component have been discussed. The discussion following each objective should be instrumental in getting you to think about how the criterion should be written to reflect how the client is expected to perform. Many of the revisions show how the criterion can be stated more clearly to avoid misinterpretation.

QUICK CHECK

There are a few important points to remember when constructing the criterion portion of a behavioral objective. Make certain the criterion is stated as accurately as possible so that it is possible to determine when the objective is accomplished.

OBJECTIVES PROBLEM 6: LACK OF SUPPORT OR HARMONY

This problem is unlike those previously discussed. Although it does not involve one of the components, it is of a more serious nature. Many of the previous problems could be identified by solely reading the behavioral objective. This problem, however, cannot be identified in this manner because the objectives are well written on the surface. Problems do not appear until the behavioral objectives are read immediately before, or during, the observation of the therapy session. Only then is it discovered that what is occurring in the therapy session does not support the objective. In other words, there is a *lack of harmony between the objective and the procedures initiated to meet that objective.* This problem frequently occurs when there is little or no direction in the client's therapy program or if no critical thought has gone into determining the objectives.

When this lack of harmony between the objective and procedure is evident, it must be decided whether the objective is correct or the procedure is correct. Based on this decision, appropriate changes must be made.

In the following examples, it was determined that what was occurring in the session was appropriate. It was also determined that the goals were not written specifically enough; therefore, they had to be revised. Although the revisions all dealt with making the performance component of the objective more specific, this problem warrants special discussion because it goes beyond merely writing the objective.

The format for this next section is first to state the behavioral objective as written by the beginning clinician. Behaviors from the therapy session are then described and discussed. A revised objective supporting the therapy session is then provided.

The first objective is:

6.1(U) to produce the /r/ phoneme correctly in sentences in 90% of his attempts

During the session, the child said *scarf* in the sentence *I have a scarf* and was reinforced for this production. According to the original goal, production of *scarf* should not be reinforced because it does not contain the consonantal /r/ phoneme. The word *scarf* contains the centering diphthong /ɑr/, which is not the same as /r/, which refers to consonantal /r/ as found in the word *red*.

After discussion with the beginning clinician, it was determined that correct production of the *centering diphthongs* was the target behavior. The goal was then revised. It is:

6.1(C) to produce <u>centering diphthongs</u> correctly in sentences in 90% of his attempts

By making the performance portion of the objective more specific, harmony was obtained between the objective and the procedure.

The second objective to be presented for discussion is:

6.2(U) to produce the /s/ phoneme correctly during conversation in 90% of his attempts

During the session, the beginning clinician reinforced the client's production of *swim*. The *sw* combination is a blend or consonant cluster and is not included in the original objective. After reading the objective, the supervisor expected the client to be reinforced for the production of /s/ in words said during conversation such as *sun, ice,* and *bicycle,* but not *swim*. Prior to the discussion with the beginning clinician, an objective to reflect the above would be:

6.2(C.1) to produce /s/ blends correctly during conversation in 90% of his attempts

Continued observation of the session revealed that the beginning clinician reinforced production of the /s/ phoneme in the words *sit* and *nest*. Discussion with the beginning clinician revealed that she viewed the goal as being correct production of the /s/ phoneme in all possible contexts. Therefore, it was necessary to revise the goal. It is:

6.2(C.2) to produce /s/ correctly in all contexts during conversation in 90% of his attempts

With the objective written in this manner, it is appropriate for the beginning clinician to reinforce correct production of /s/ as singletons, blends, or sound combinations. Harmony now exists between the objective and the procedure. This harmony was accomplished by making the performance portion of the objective more specific.

The next objective to be examined is:

6.3(U) to produce the /s/ phoneme correctly during reading in 90% of his attempts

The client's production of the words *bees* and *was* was reinforced during the reading activity. Both of these words end in the /z/ phoneme and therefore are not included in the original objective.

After discussion with the beginning clinician, it was learned that she was looking for correct production of both members of the cognate pair. This information should have been reflected in the objective. Therefore, a revised objective is:

6.3(C) to produce the /s/ and /z/ phonemes correctly during reading in 90% of his attempts

The objective is now supported by the procedure. Once again, harmony was achieved by making the performance portion of the objective more specific.

In summary, the three examples cited in this section all involve what appear to be well-written behavioral objectives. The three components (performance, condition, and criterion) are intact—at least at first glance. When the therapy session is observed concurrent with reading the objectives, a lack of harmony between the objective and the procedure becomes evident. In the examples cited, harmony was achieved by making the performance aspect of the objective more specific.

QUICK CHECK

Always make certain there is harmony between your objectives and procedures. Make certain that all of your procedures support your objectives.

CONCLUSION

This chapter shows various problems that arise in writing behavioral objectives. The first problem, incorrect format following the lead-in, deals with lack of consistency between the lead-in and the actual objective. Problems two through five deal with the performance, condition, or criterion component of the behavioral objective. The last, lack of support or harmony, deals with the lack of agreement between the objective and the procedure. Now that these common problems have been identified, it is hoped that you will give more analytic and critical thought to your behavioral objectives before submitting them to your clinical supervisor.

KNOW IT! USE IT!

After reading this chapter, you should be able to:

1. state at least three problems affecting the performance component of behavioral objectives
2. explain the main problem affecting the condition component of behavioral objectives
3. state at least three problems affecting the criterion component of behavioral objectives
4. write at least four problem-free behavioral objectives reflecting four different communication disorders
5. detect and fix all problems evident in your behavioral objectives

REFERENCE

Van Riper, C., & Emerick, L. (1990). *Speech correction: An introduction to speech pathology and audiology.* Englewood Cliffs, NJ: Prentice-Hall.

CHAPTER 3

Evaluations and Progress Reports: Organization and Content

CHAPTER HIGHLIGHTS

- *critically analyzing evaluations*
- *content to include in evaluations*
- *organization of evaluations*
- *problems to avoid while writing evaluations*
- *developing a sense for writing evaluations*
- *content to include in progress reports*
- *organization of progress reports*
- *developing a sense for writing progress notes*

The format and content of an evaluation vary depending on the professional setting in which it is prepared, as well as on the disorder exhibited. In this chapter, the need for writing professional evaluations will be demonstrated by first presenting a poorly written example. This evaluation, written by a clinician with a master's degree, came across my desk many years ago. I saved it because it was so unique. It has been presented to many beginning clinicians as their first exposure to analyzing an evaluation critically. You will see that it is a challenge to determine what is wrong and to suggest improvements. Because all of your reports and evaluations remain in client files long after you have prepared them, it is extremely important to develop good professional writing skills. This topic will again come to light, and be given added meaning, in our discussion of accountability.

SUBSTANDARD EVALUATION

All you know now is that this evaluation is substandard. You might, however, read it and wonder **why** it is unacceptable. If that is the case, do not worry. Reread the example (Exhibit 3–1) and ask yourself, "Does this clearly and completely describe the client's condition and the proposed actions? Is it well organized and clearly written?" Then read the analysis which follows.

Exhibit 3–1 Speech and Language Evaluation Report

Sally A. Smith
000 Main Street
Snowtown, PA 00000
D.O.B. 0/0/00
Foster parents: Betty and Bill Brown

This is a three year-2 month old girl who is seen for a speech and language evaluation at the request of Snowtown's County Children's Services. Mary Doe is the caseworker. It is felt that she is delayed in speech and language acquisition for her age. The history is quite involved. She was taken into a foster home at the age of 18 months. At that time, she was said to be deprived and almost in a catatonic state. She didn't talk at all and didn't smile. It took several weeks for the foster parents to get her to smile and at 23 months of age she said "mommy".

Up until the age of 18 months, it was felt that Sally was on a very poor diet. She was taken care of at times by a half sister. Her mother died when she was 13 months old. Informally, it has been ascertained that the mother's health was quite poor during pregnancy. The cause of death was a stroke so we might get some hint of some of the problems that she had from this. Evidently the home situation was terrible.

She has been seen at Snowtown Medical Center and they have stated that she has delayed bone age. However, according to the foster mother, she has been progressing nicely as of late. The foster mother seems to be quite quick to explain Sally's slowness as functional and is quite adamant about the fact that she is not retarded. At present, she is beginning to put words together. Her intelligibility is quite poor. Therefore, I could not obtain much in the way of an articulation sample. I was able to obtain a raw score on Form A of the Peabody Picture Vocabulary Test. This was 12, which converts to a mental age of 2–3, an intelligence quotient of 73 and a percentile score of 2. The reliability of these tests at the low end of the age spectrum is quite poor, and therefore the score is certainly no better than a ball park score. It is felt that Sally has not had any ear infections and that she can hear well. The hearing screening that we did was essentially normal.

Certainly, from the history that we obtained, it seems as though we are dealing with a case of delayed speech and language acquisition that may certainly be explained in part or in its entirety by the very poor situation in which this child found herself for the first 18 months of her life during which the linguistic foundation should have been built. She will be attending a nursery program at Snowtown College and it would seem as though it would be most convenient for the parent if her speech therapy session could be plugged in to this. Therefore, I will be contacting Mrs.

continues

Exhibit 3–1 continued

White of Snowtown College Speech Dept. to see if she will be able to work this out. If this is not possible then we could consider seeing Sally down here for speech therapy, but in view of the convenience of the college to the parents I would suggest that they try to work it in up there.

I would like to see Sally back here in about six months for further speech evaluation.

_____
(name)

cc: Mary Doe, SCCS [Snowtown's County Children's Services]
Mrs. White, Speech Dept. Snowtown College

ANALYSIS

Although this might be an acceptable style for a social history evaluation, it is poorly organized for a speech and language evaluation. Information needs to be organized by topic rather than appearing at various places throughout the evaluation. Headings and subheadings should be used to organize the information and to assist the reader in locating information. Simple information, such as a telephone number for the foster parents is missing, making it difficult to contact them.

To help you understand the problems, the following topics will be used to review this evaluation: background information, clinical assessment, writing style, and grammar. Although no priority is implied by this order, you will later be shown an organizational outline to use in your reports and be given instructions on how to use language to convey your thoughts accurately. Keep in mind that these problems were unique to the person who wrote this evaluation. You may have other weaknesses, such as use of poor grammar and/or poor writing skills, that you can start to work on immediately.

Background Information: Descriptive Data

Source

Certain data are basic to these reports and are included because they aid comprehension. Here, it is not known from where the evaluator obtained the information in the first two paragraphs and at the beginning of the third. Mary Doe is cited as the caseworker, but it does not state that she provided any background information. It is not known whether the caseworker accompanied the child to the evaluation. After reading, "It is felt that she is delayed in speech and language acquisition for her age," one wonders who initially felt that a delay was evident. It is not known who diagnosed delayed bone age at the Snowtown Medical Center. It is mentioned in the evaluation that the foster mother is adamant about Sally not being retarded, but, again, the source of the information is not known. Was it related by the caseworker or the foster mother herself? Was the foster mother present? Was the information provided on a case history intake form and, if so, who completed it? Likewise, the source is not known for the following statement: "It is felt that Sally has not had any ear infections and that she can hear well."

Dates

The evaluation does not provide the date of this report, the date on which Sally was seen at the Snowtown Medical Center, or how old she was when delayed bone age was diagnosed. Likewise, it is not possible to determine when Sally's mother suffered the stroke or when she passed away. It is important to know how old Sally was at the time of these devastating events.

Social and Developmental History

These data must be presented in some logical order or sequence. Looking at the ages stated, for example one sees 18 months, 23 months, 18 months, and then 13 months. It would be easier to follow if the information were presented in a chronological fashion.

Unsupported Statements

All statements should be documented. In other words, there should be information in the evaluation that leads to each statement. For example, after reading, "Up until the age of 18 months, it was felt that Sally was on a very poor diet," one asks why? What information was presented to lead to this statement? Nowhere in this evaluation was information presented to support this statement. Additional examples are "Informally, it has been ascertained that the mother's health was quite poor during pregnancy" and "Evidently the home situation was terrible." Many of these statements are not based on fact. There is no information provided in the evaluation that forms the basis for these statements.

Clinical Assessment

Objectives

After performing an evaluation, one should know exactly at what level the child is functioning in the area(s) of speech and/or language, at what level the child should be functioning given his or her chronological age or mental age, and the best path to help him or her get there. We know that this path is a series of small steps called objectives. At the end of an evaluation report, the immediate objectives of therapy should be stated. They are absent, however, in this evaluation.

Diagnoses

The evaluator states that Sally has delayed speech, but this diagnosis is not supported in the body of the report. The only statements pertaining to her speech are "Her intelligibility is quite poor" and "Therefore, I could not obtain much in the way of an articulation sample." Solely on the basis of these two statements, the diagnosis of delayed speech was made. There is nothing specific known about the child's speech. Additional information should be included. Among others, information such as phonemes the child can produce correctly, substituted phonemes and the nature of the substitution, omitted phonemes, vowel production, stimulability, and phonological processes are essential pieces of information that should be included in an evaluation. If this information were provided, perhaps the diagnosis of delayed speech could be supported.

The evaluator also states that the child has delayed language. A statement was made that "she is beginning to put words together" and that she had "a percentile score of 2" on the *Peabody Picture Vocabulary Test.* Although two statements about the child's language are made, the diagnosis is weakly supported, and the child's present level of language functioning is still not known. Much more relevant information should have been included in the evaluation. All relevant aspects of language should have been addressed. For example, the following information would be helpful: how many different single words does the child use, how many two-word utterances does the child use and what type(s) (agent + action, action + object, agent + object, etc.), and overall how does the child communicate her wants and needs? In addition, pragmatics and semantics were not addressed thoroughly.

Writing Style and Grammar

Precision and Clarity in Word Selection

The vocabulary chosen should be precise, clear, and appropriate for professional writing. If it is not, the evaluation will lose some or all of its validity. Examples of substandard vocabulary selection can be seen in the underlinings in the following examples: "The reliability of these tests at the low end of the age spectrum is quite poor, and therefore the score is certainly no better than a <u>ball park</u> score. . . . She will be attending a nursery program at Snowtown College and it would seem as though it would be most convenient for the parent if her speech therapy session could be <u>plugged</u> in to [into] this. . . . If this is not possible then we could consider seeing Sally <u>down here</u> for speech therapy, but in view of the convenience of the college to the parents I would suggest that they try to work it in <u>up there</u>. . . . I would like to see Sally <u>back here</u> in about six months for further speech evaluation." The underlined word selections are not evident of good vocabulary selection for professional evaluations. Many of them are too colloquial for professional writing.

Use of Pronouns

Pronouns have a tendency to confuse readers unless the referent for each pronoun is obvious. It should not be necessary to search previous text to determine the referent of a pronoun. Referents that are not clear lead to ambiguity and inaccuracy. For example, let us look at some sentences from the original evaluation. "Mary Doe is the caseworker. It is felt that she is delayed in speech and language acquisition for her age." The referent *she* pertains to Mary Doe; however it is Sally A. Smith who has the speech and language delay. "She was *taken* into a foster home at the age of 18 months" also incorrectly refers to the caseworker and not the client. This referent problem continues throughout the first paragraph. Other examples are "At that time, she was said to be deprived and almost in a catatonic state," and "*She* didn't talk at all and didn't smile." In addition to a problem with the pronoun *she* in the next example, there is a problem with the pronoun *her,* as both referents imply the caseworker when they are supposed to pertain to the client. The example is, "It took several weeks for the foster parents to get *her* to smile and at 23 months of age she said "mommy". In the second paragraph, it is confusing as to whose mother died because in the sentence "*Her* mother died when she was 13 months old," the referent for both *her* and *she* is *half sister*. The next sentence is also problematic. It is, "The cause of death was a stroke so we might get some hint of some of the problems that *she* had from this." Once again, the referent is inaccurate. The last-mentioned noun was "mother," but it appears that the evaluator's intent is to refer to Sally. The intent is not clear. The next example is found in the first sentence of the third paragraph which starts with a pronoun. It is, "*She* has been seen at Snowtown Medical Center and *they* have stated that she has delayed bone age." The last referent mentioned was "mother" in the sentence, "Informally, it has been ascertained that the mother's health was quite poor during pregnancy." Another referent problem with the sentence concerns the pronoun *they.* The person(s) who diagnosed delayed bone age was never mentioned and the "center" itself does not diagnose. Notice that "she" is used three times in the third paragraph before the introduction of any referent, and each is ambiguous.

Contractions. Contractions are not generally acceptable in formal writing and are out of place except when used to cite specific examples of sentences used by the client. There are two examples of contraction usage in the evaluation being analyzed. They are, "She *didn't* talk at all and *didn't* smile."

Abbreviations. As a general principle, abbreviations should not be used in formal writing. The sole example in the evaluation is "Therefore, I will be contacting Mrs. White of Snowtown College Speech Dept. to see if she will be able to work this out."

There are exceptions to this principle that pertain to technical writing in which abbreviations of lengthy technical terminology are more easily recognized than the terms themselves. When a term is abbreviated, however, it must be spelled out completely the first time it appears and then must be followed immediately by its abbreviation in parentheses. Thereafter, the abbreviation can be used in text without further explanation. An example not based on the evaluation is "The **Peabody Picture Vocabulary Test—Revised (PPVT)** was administered to determine functioning in receptive vocabulary."

First- or Third-Person Writing Style

Problems are evident with writing both in the first and third persons. It is best to avoid using first person in an evaluation. Referring to yourself as "I" comes across as trying to increase your importance. Likewise, reference to yourself in the third person as "the evaluator" is somewhat ambiguous and can give the impression of trying to deny your findings. Examples of first-person usage from Exhibit 3–1 are "Therefore, *I* could not obtain much in the way of an articulation sample. *I* was able to obtain a raw score on Form A of the **Peabody Picture Vocabulary Test**. . . . Therefore, *I* will be contacting Mrs. White of Snowtown College Speech Dept. to see whether she will be able to work this out. If this is not possible then we would consider seeing Sally down here for speech therapy, but in view of the convenience of the college to the parents, *I* would suggest that they try to work it in up there. *I* would like to see Sally back here in about six months for further speech evaluation."

One way to avoid using first-person pronouns is to switch from active voice to passive voice. However, active is the preferable voice because it is more forceful and direct. Suggestions for changing the examples provided in order to avoid using first person are "Therefore, it was difficult to obtain an articulation sample"; "A raw score of 12 was obtained on the **Peabody Picture Vocabulary Test**"; "Therefore, Mrs. White of Snowtown College Speech Department will be contacted to see if she can make suitable arrangements. If suitable arrangements cannot be made at Snowtown College, Sally will be scheduled to receive services at this facility. Because of the convenience for the parents if services were rendered at the College, it is strongly suggested that this avenue be pursued. Sally's speech and language should be reevaluated at this facility in 6 months."

The evaluation being analyzed did not contain usage of third person in the sense just described here. However, this problem can also be rectified in the same manner as in the first person example by using passive voice.

The third-person plural pronoun "we" should not have been used because the work was done by one person. One person performed the evaluation, and that same person wrote the evaluation report. Therefore, the use of "we" in these contexts is misleading. Examples of "we" usage in the evaluation being analyzed are "The hearing screening that _we_ did was essentially normal. Certainly, from the history that _we_ obtained, it seems as though we are dealing with a case of delayed speech and language acquisition that may certainly be explained in part or in its entirety by the very poor situation in which this child found herself for the first 18 months of her life during which the linguistic foundation should have been built. . . . If this is not possible then _we_ could consider seeing Sally down here for speech therapy, but in view of the convenience of the college to the parents I would suggest that they try to work it in up there."

QUICK CHECK

Now that you have experience critically analyzing evaluations, use this information to analyze your evaluations. Make certain your house is in order!

GENERAL GUIDELINES FOR SPEECH-LANGUAGE EVALUATIONS

Evaluations must be of professional caliber because they will be sent to other agencies or professionals. To help you get a good start with the writing process, general guidelines are now presented. It must be understood that these are merely _guidelines_ and _may_ have to be modified to meet the needs of each client, the format of the facility, or your supervisor's preferred format. The following content areas should be included when a child's speech and language are being evaluated and can be presented in the order shown (identifying information, background information, evaluation, impressions, and recommendations). Evaluations should use headings and subheadings to assist with organization and should contain the following information if appropriate. Headings and subheadings should be either underlined, boldfaced, or italicized for easy identification.

The heading *identifying information* does not overtly appear on written evaluations, although the actual information is presented. It is obvious what this information is and thus does not need to be identified with a heading. This heading is used in Exhibit 4–1 in brackets solely to emphasize organization through the use of headings.

There is no one standard model used for speech-language evaluations. There are, however, two formats, and a variation of the one, that seem to be used more frequently than others. In one format, paragraphs are indented and an extra space exists between the paragraphs under the same heading. A variation of this format, used in chapter 4, occurs when paragraphs are likewise indented but an extra space does not exist between paragraphs under the same heading. Another format frequently used follows block style in which paragraphs are not indented and an extra space exists between paragraphs addressing the same heading.

What about length? Most beginning clinicians want to know how long an evaluation needs to be. As has always been true, there is no magic number of pages. Evaluations must cover all the basic information and then some. Exactly "how much" is a function of the nature of the client's involvement, as well as the clinician's knowledge and ability to focus on important information.

[Identifying Information]

The following information should be presented in the manner shown:

NAME:	FILE NUMBER:
ADDRESS:	EVALUATION DATE:
	BIRTHDATE:
PHONE	AGE:
PARENTS: (if applicable)	STUDENT CLINICIAN:
	SEMESTER:

The format for this section may vary among settings. Categories such as "referral source," "school/preschool," "family physician," and "problem" might be required in some settings. A good rule of thumb is to familiarize yourself with the format used in your setting before writing your first evaluation.

The "age" category needs some explanation. If the client is a child, the exact age in years and months should be provided. For example, if a child's age is 3 years, 1 month, and 21 days, an age of 3 years, 2 months should be stated. Generally, if a child is older than 15 days, an extra month is added. Further, once a child reaches adolescence, it usually is not necessary to state the age in years and months. This is because there is no difference in speech, language, or communication functioning between, for example, age 14 years, 0 months and 14 years, 11 months. However, an exception must be made if a particular test administered differentiates between various months of a particular age. If this is the case, it is necessary to provide the age in years and months.

Background Information

The information to be obtained for this section will vary pending the age and condition of the client. This section should include the reason the person is being evaluated, as well as the source of referral. If the client is self-referred or parent-referred, the reason for referral should be stated using the client's or parent's words as appropriate.

If the client was previously enrolled in therapy, state where therapy was obtained. Provide the name of the clinician if possible. Summarize the therapeutic objectives if the informant can provide this information. State when therapy began and when it was terminated. State the reason for termination.

If the client is a child, speech and language milestones (age at which the first word was spoken, what the first word was, age at which two-word utterances were spoken, etc.) should be included. If the child is not yet producing two-word utterances, state how large the child's vocabulary is. If the child is not yet using words, state how he or she gets his or her wants and needs across.

Developmental milestones should be included for young children. At what age did the child perform the following: sit with support, move by creeping, sit easily unsupported, crawl, pull himself or herself up to a standing position, take stepping movements, take the first independent step, walk when one hand was held, walk with feet slightly apart without falling, walk upstairs unassisted, walk up and downstairs alone without alternating steps, walk upstairs alternating feet, become toilet trained during the day, and become toilet trained during the day and night. Only include information pertaining to those milestones that should have been mastered previously.

Birth history should be reported, but, again, areas to emphasize will vary pending each client. It might be important to obtain information about the following: the length of pregnancy, the child's birth weight, hazards present (Was labor induced?), the mother's health during pregnancy, the duration of labor, type of delivery (vaginal, breech, or cesarean section), instruments used during delivery if applicable, incubation at birth and how long if applicable, color of the child at birth, scars or bruises present at birth, the length of time it took the child to regain birth weight, and whether the child had difficulty sucking.

Medical history should be included. Inquire about the client's general health and what diseases he or she has had. Find out whether the child ever had a high fever and, if so, ask if he ever had convulsions.

Additional information is needed if the client is an adult. It is important to include the client's educational and vocational history.

If much of this information appears in previous evaluations done at either another or the present facility, state the significant information as well as new information in your evaluation. To refer the reader to another evaluation, state, "Additional background information may be found in the May [include applicable year] evaluation done at _____ [state the complete name of the facility]," if performed at another facility or, "Additional background information may be found in the Spring [include applicable year] evaluation," if performed at the same facility.

In general, it will be up to you to determine the actual organization of the "Background Information" section. If you have a lot of information for particular aspects (previous therapy, speech and language milestones, developmental milestones, etc.), the use of subheadings will be helpful for organizational purposes. If you do not have a lot of information, the use of new paragraphs for each aspect will be adequate.

Evaluation

This section should contain some brief introductory information that will "set the tone." Examples are "John performed all tasks willingly and interacted well with the examiner. He was quite verbal and appeared to be unaware of any communication difficulty," "John was very cooperative at the beginning of the evaluation. After 20 minutes, his attention was lost and he could not be directed back to tasks," "Sally willingly separated from her mother and eagerly entered the evaluation room. She was extremely verbal and attempted all tasks enthusiastically," "John performed all tasks willingly and interacted well with the examiner during the evaluation. It was noted, however, that he asked to have numerous items repeated on the various tests administered during the evaluation," and "John clung to his mother and tears welled in his eyes when the examiner extended her hand to lead him to the evaluation room. It was then decided that he should be accompanied by his mother, who remained present throughout the evaluation. With his mother present, John was cooperative and attempted all tasks."

Speech

State the name of the test(s) administered and what the test(s) measures. Provide scores and their interpretation. If the client exhibits an articulation problem, results can be reported by listing the findings in terms of omissions, substitutions, distortions, and additions. Include the position(s) in which the error(s) occurred. After analysis, state whether any entire phoneme class is in error. State which phonemes the child should have already mastered according to norms (those accompanying the test administered, Sander (1972), Lowe (1986), or Prather, Hedrick & Kern (1975), etc.). The norm used should be cited. If a client exhibits a phonological process problem, indicate the phonological processes present. Provide examples for all existing processes.

In addition to the client's single-word production, evaluate his speech informally during conversation. Determine whether the client's articulatory performance on single words is similar to his performance in conversation. Determine the client's percentage of intelligibility. Include a statement about the consistency of errors, the stimulability of the misarticulated sounds, and the highest level at which the client had success, if any, on errored phonemes (isolation, syllables, word, phrase, etc.). If the client has a problem, indicate whether he showed signs of awareness. If any errors are conspicuous, a description and explanation should be provided.

Fluency and Rate

If it is obvious that the client has disfluencies and if this is the reason that he or she is being evaluated, a different evaluation format should be followed. Disfluencies will be analyzed in detail, and it probably will not be necessary to look at speech and language in depth.

If the client has "normal nonfluencies," explain the nonfluencies but indicate that they are to be expected for his age. If the client's fluency is within normal limits, so state.

If uncertain as to whether the client's rate is within normal limits, tape record a 1-minute sample of conversational speech. Count the number of words produced in 1 minute. A normal speaking rate is approximately 175 words per minute.

Language

Receptive Ability

State which test(s) was administered and state what was assessed (receptive vocabulary, etc.). State the results of each test and include the receptive language age if applicable. If there is a delay, state the length of the delay. Be certain to include areas in which the client successfully performed, as well as areas in which the client experienced difficulty. In other words, summarize the client's performance.

Go beyond formal tests. Determine whether the client understands conversation. Provide evidence. Additional ideas of areas to explore will be presented. However, it will be necessary to use your professional judgment to determine which aspects of receptive language should be pursued for each individual client. It is also possible that many of these aspects were incorporated into the formal test(s) which was administered. If this is the case, there is no need to "test" them again. You may want to include some of the following information in your evaluation if pertinent. Does the client follow simple directions, understand basic concepts, identify common objects, identify body parts, identify common objects when their use is given, match colors, understand prepositions, and understand size (big and little) and quality (more and less)?

Expressive Ability

This section should address syntax, morphology, semantics, and pragmatics. State which test(s) was administered and state what was assessed. State the results of each test and include the expressive language age. If there is a delay, state the length of the delay. Include areas in which the client successfully performed, as well as areas of difficulty. Evaluate the client's language informally and formally. Overall, summarize the client's performance.

Oral Peripheral Examination

The oral peripheral examination should be performed toward the end of your evaluation. In this manner, you have the opportunity to observe the structural design as well as its function as the client is communicating and performing other tasks. Directly assess only those structures or functions that are suspect as a result of your observations.

It is recommended that the two main aspects, *structure* and *function,* be discussed separately. It is not enough to state that the structure and function are within normal limits. It is necessary to state specifically the findings on which this conclusion of normalcy is based.

Structure

Examine the client's lips to determine whether they are of normal size, shape, and symmetry. Examine the relationship of the mandible to the maxilla. Ascertain whether the occlusion is normal. Examine the client's tongue and determine whether it is of normal shape, size, and symmetry. Examine the hard and soft palates.

Function

Determine whether the client can protrude and retract his lips. See if this can be done in quick succession. Ascertain whether the client can elevate, depress, protrude, retract, and lateralize his tongue. Determine whether there is adequate velopharyngeal closure on the production of /ɑ/. Check the client's diadochokinesis.

Vocal Parameters

If the client's main complaint is not one dealing with voice, informally assess this aspect. Listen to the client during conversation. If his voice appears to be normal, state "the vocal parameters were informally assessed during conversation. Pitch, quality, and loudness were within normal limits for (name's) age, gender, and size." If, however, the client does have a voice problem, the parameters of pitch, quality, and loudness must be thoroughly evaluated, and the contents of the evaluation presented would be altered because it is probable that the client's speech and language would not need to be thoroughly evaluated.

Auditory Sensitivity

Conduct a pure-tone hearing screening test. State that a pure-tone hearing screening test was administered to assess (name's) hearing sensitivity. State the frequencies tested and the decibel (dB) level used. Usually, the following frequencies are tested in each ear: 250, 500, 1000, 2000, and 4000 Hz. A 25 dB level is usually used. State the conditions in which the testing occurred (quiet, noisy, etc.). State whether the client passed the screening in both ears, in the right ear, or in the left ear. State how the client indicated that he heard the tone.

It appears appropriate at this point to discuss an ethical issue regarding the use of audiometry in clinical practice by speech-language-certified persons who are not certified in audiology. The position of the American Speech-Language-Hearing Association (ASHA) is:

> Individuals who hold only the CCC-SLP may perform or supervise pure tone air conduction hearing screening procedures for persons who can reliably participate in such procedures through conditioned play or con-

ventional behavioral responses. The screening procedures employed shall be developed in consultation with an individual holding the CCC-A and shall be in compliance with current applicable ASHA policies. Individuals who hold the CCC-SLP shall limit judgments and descriptive statements about the results of hearing screening procedures to whether the person has passed or failed the screening. Persons who fail the hearing screening should be referred to a certified audiologist. (American Speech-Language-Hearing Association, 1991, p. 51)

The bottom line is that it is unethical for a speech-language pathologist to perform a threshold test. Speech-language pathologists are only qualified to perform hearing screening tests and are only allowed to state whether a person *passed* or *failed.* It is not ethical to interpret the findings in any other way.

Impressions

This section follows from the rest of the written evaluation. *Information for which the groundwork has not been done does not belong in this section.* The nature and severity of the client's speech and/or language problem is stated in this section and should be based on the analysis of formal and informal test results and the client's history, along with observations of the client and his parents (if applicable). This is the point at which the information is interpreted. In other words, state what the information means. A statement summarizing areas of normal functioning should also be included. Prognosis for improvement and the basis for this prediction should be stated in this section. The type of problem and severity likewise belongs here.

Recommendations

Make certain that the reader has previously been provided with an adequate basis for understanding the recommendations made in this section. General and specific recommendations should be stated. An example is as follows:
It is recommended that:

1. (Name) receive language therapy on a twice a week basis
2. (Name) receive a thorough audiological examination to determine current hearing acuity
3. language therapy should emphasize production of two-word utterances

Please note that if you are not going to be providing the therapeutic services, it is best not to recommend particular tests or programs to be used with the client, as the clinician who will be providing the services may have individual preferences or limited access to materials.

[Signatures]

The heading *signatures* does not overtly appear on evaluations, although the section is present. Once again, it is obvious what the *signatures* are and thus does not need to be identified with a heading. However, this heading is used here in brackets solely to emphasize the organizational structure of an evaluation. At the conclusion of an evaluation, you and your supervisor need to sign it. It is neither necessary nor appropriate to include your institutional affiliation, as this will be obvious from the letterhead stationery on which it is prepared.

Jane Doe
Jane Doe
Undergraduate Student Clinician

Betty A. Brown, M.S. CCC/SLP
Betty A. Brown, M.S. CCC/SLP
Clinical Supervisor

> **QUICK CHECK**
>
> Upon completion of your evaluations, make certain you have adequately addressed all the necessary content areas. Make certain headings and sub-headings are used appropriately.

PROGRESS REPORTS/ORGANIZATION AND CONTENT

As therapy progresses, it is necessary to learn to write another type of report, a progress report. These reports must also be written in a professional manner. This will not be as monumental a task as writing evaluations because many aspects of writing evaluations will be incorporated into writing progress reports.

Progress reports are written for clients who have been receiving therapy in order to document any improvement that has been made. Progress reports are usually written at the end of each semester. In this manner, the clinician who will be assigned to the client the following semester will have a good idea of what has been done, as well as where to begin. Examples of progress reports can be found in chapter 4.

GENERAL GUIDELINES FOR SPEECH-LANGUAGE PROGRESS REPORTS

Progress reports, like evaluations, must be of professional caliber because they will also be sent to other agencies or professionals. Please keep in mind that the guidelines presented here will have to be modified to meet the needs of each client. The following content areas should be included and can be presented in the order provided. Progress reports should use headings and subheadings to assist with organization and should contain the following information if appropriate. Headings and subheadings should be underlined, boldfaced, or italicized for easy identification.

[Identifying Information]

The following information should be provided:

NAME:	FILE NUMBER:
ADDRESS:	DATE:
	BIRTHDATE:
PHONE:	AGE:
PARENTS: (if applicable)	STUDENT CLINICIAN:
	SEMESTER:

Background Information

In sentence form, state the client's name and exact age in years and months if appropriate. State the exact name of the facility at which therapy was received. State the client's original diagnosis and include the severity and date at the time of the diagnosis. State the client's diagnosis and severity when last evaluated. Include the number of sessions the client attended of the possible number he could have attended. Include the dates (beginning and ending) of these sessions. Any additional information that has not been included in one of the previous evaluations or progress reports should be noted in this section.

Additional Testing (optional)

This section will be included if any additional testing was done after the evaluation was completed but during the same semester. Because the results of this testing could not be included in the evaluation, they should be covered in this section. Frequently, tests that were administered at the beginning of the semester as part of the initial evaluation are administered again at the end of the semester as another attempt to measure progress. In this case, the results of the both tests should be cited as well as compared.

Therapeutic Objectives

List the objectives for the current semester. Use this format:

The objectives for this semester were:

1. _____

2. _____

Progress and Procedures

Address each objective individually. Summarize the actual procedure used to achieve each objective. Vary the lead-ins. An example is "Objective one (correct production of the /s/ phoneme in isolation) was accomplished by using a combination of phonetic placement and auditory stimulation." Briefly explain these techniques. Do not state the materials used, as they are *not* a part of the procedure. Another example is "To accomplish objective one (receptive identification of verbs). . . ." Indicate progress, if made, by using percentages or some other objective measurement. Be certain to state the client's level of performance at the beginning of the semester and at the end of the semester. For example, "At the beginning of the semester, John could not correctly produce the /s/ phoneme in isolation. He currently produces it correctly in 80% of his attempts." It would also be acceptable to include in this section activities that the client liked or specific techniques used to help control unwanted behaviors.

Current Status and Impressions

State the current diagnosis and compare it with the original diagnosis. Include the current severity of the problem(s). Include the prognosis for further improvement if indicated. Provide support for this prognosis.

Recommendations

State whether therapy should be continued the next semester or if it should be terminated. State whether or not the client should be re-evaluated the next semester. State objectives for the next semester, if applicable, in this manner: "Pending a re-evaluation in the (spring or fall) semester, possible therapeutic objectives are. . . ." Be specific, but it is not necessary to state criterion at this time.

[Signatures]

Jane Doe
_____
Jane Doe
Undergraduate Student Clinician

Betty A. Brown, M.S. CCC/SLP
_____
Betty A. Brown, M.S. CCC/SLP
Clinical Supervisor

QUICK CHECK

When writing progress reports, be certain to include the necessary content areas. Use appropriate headings and subheadings to assist with your organization.

KNOW IT! USE IT!

After reading this chapter, you should be able to:

1. state at least five problems found in the "substandard" evaluation
2. state five content areas (headings) to include in a speech and language evaluation
3. state at least two general pieces of information to be included under each of the five content areas in a speech and language evaluation
4. state at least five problems to avoid while writing evaluations
5. state seven content areas (headings) that may be included in a speech-language progress report
6. state at least two general pieces of information to be included under each of the seven content areas (headings) in a speech-language progress report

REFERENCES

American Speech-Language-Hearing Association. (1991). Issues in ethics: Clinical practice by certificate holders in the profession in which they are not certified. *Asha, 33*(12), 51.

Lowe, R. (1986). *Assessment link between phonology and articulation (ALPHA)*. East Moline, IL: Linguisystems.

Prather, E., Hedrick, D., & Kern, C. (1975). Articulation development in children aged two to four years. *Journal of Speech and Hearing Disorders, 40*(2), 179–191.

Sander, E. (1972). When are speech sounds learned? *Journal of Speech and Hearing Disorders, 37*(1), 55–63.

CHAPTER 4

Evaluations, Re-Evaluations, and Progress Reports: Writing Reports That Shine

CHAPTER HIGHLIGHTS

- *develop a deeper sense for writing evaluations*
- *develop a sense for writing re-evaluations*
- *develop a deeper sense for writing progress reports*

This chapter contains samples of evaluations, re-evaluations, and progress reports that can be considered well written. It is inevitable that some speech-language pathology supervisors will have comments on how to improve these or other evaluations, re-evaluations, or progress reports by changing them to reflect their own styles. This only means that there is a zone of acceptance for professional reports, and no single or best way to write professional reports can be offered. There are, however, a few basic guidelines that should be kept in mind when writing professional reports. According to Paul-Brown (1994, p. 41),

"Writing should be clearly understood by the reader; that is, content should be:

1. accurate, concise, and informative
2. adapted for a potentially large readership
3. useful and relevant to other staff (i.e., so that anyone can pick up record and continue treatment)
4. neat and legible."

If these points are followed, written material will be completed with a minimum number of rewrites and the final document will both contain pertinent content and be easy to read.

One way to get a feel or sense for the flow and style of professional writing is to read and reread samples written by other professionals. The documents in this chapter will provide you with a springboard into this process as you analyze the meaning and word choices, as well as the sentence structures, used. Attend to the format. Observe that in these reports, paragraphs are indented but a space does not exist between paragraphs.

EVALUATIONS—SAMPLES

Evaluation One: Articulation

Exhibit 4–1 reflects an evaluation in which faulty articulation is evident. Therefore, that is the area where the most time and attention are given. Formal assessment of the child's language ability is not necessary, as problems are not evident in this area. [Note: "Identifying Information" appears in brackets throughout this chapter because this heading is not usually present in these reports. Also, references to "this year" and "last year" appear in the identifying information and background information sections. In actual evaluations, the exact year would be cited.]

Evaluation Two: Language

This evaluation (Exhibit 4–2) differs from the first evaluation in that background information must be obtained from the client's previous files. The major focus is in the area of language. The findings between informal and formal language assessment are contradictory. The manner in which this contradiction is handled is interesting.

Evaluation Three: Language and Articulation

This evaluation (Exhibit 4–3) is lengthy owing to the clinician's thoroughness and to the extent of the child's problem. The clinician's thoroughness is evident in the background information section, which is quite comprehensive, and also in the way the language sample was analyzed and interpreted. The area of pragmatics is addressed. This child exhibits a problem in receptive language, expressive language, and articulation.

Evaluation Four: Fluency

Because the focus of this evaluation (Exhibit 4–4) is fluency, speech and language do not necessarily have to be evaluated or included. The inclusion of speech and language varies according to the facility. Some facilities require that an informal statement be included for each speech or language area. If, however, a problem

Exhibit 4–1 Sample Evaluation

[Identifying Information]

NAME:	Mary Smith	FILE NUMBER:	
ADDRESS:	00 Broad Street	EVALUATION DATE:	February 4, [this year]
	Maintown, PA	BIRTHDATE:	December 9, [5 years ago]
PHONE:	000-000-0000	AGE:	4 years, 2 months
PARENTS:	Mary and Bill	CLINICIAN:	Sally Doe
PROBLEM:	Articulation	SEMESTER:	Fall [last year]

SPEECH-LANGUAGE EVALUATION

Background Information

Mary, age 4 years, 2 months, was seen for a speech evaluation on February 4 of this year after being referred by Alice Allan, a speech-language pathologist, at the Maintown Hospital and Medical Center. Ms. Allan performed a speech and language screening. Mary failed the speech screening. According to Ms. Allan, Mary's errors consisted of /f, s, ʃ, p, t, k/. Mary's mother accompanied her and served as informant. When asked to describe the problem, Mrs. Smith stated that "Mary is difficult to understand at times."

According to Mrs. Smith, Mary started using sentences at 2½ years of age. Mrs. Smith was not able to provide other speech and language milestones. Developmental milestones include sitting alone at 7 months, crawling at 7 months, standing at 11 months, walking at 1 year, feeding herself with a spoon at 16 months, toilet trained during the day at 2 years, 8 months, and toilet trained at night at 3½ years.

Mrs. Smith stated that she had no problems with her pregnancy, but she could not provide specific information such as the length of labor or her daughter's birth weight. Regarding medical history, Mary has not had any recent illnesses, injuries, or operations. She had the flu at 3 years of age and chicken pox at 3½ years of age.

Evaluation

Mary was very shy in that she hid behind her mother when it was time to separate from her and enter the testing room. She was able to be coaxed. Mary was very soft spoken throughout the evaluation. She cooperated and performed all tasks.

continues

Exhibit 4–1 continued

Speech

The **Arizona Articulation Proficiency Scale** was administered to assess articulation on single words. The results were:

Omissions	Substitutions	Distortions
h (I)	b/f (I)	None
t (F)	g/k (I)	
ks (F)	d/j (I)	
ts (F)	b/p (I)	
	d/t (I)	
	w/v (I)	
	b/v (F)	
	w/r (I)	
	t/θ (I)	
	d/ð (I)	
	t/ʃ (F)	
	d/z (I,F)	
	d/s (I)	
	t/s (F)	
	b/pl (I)	
	t/tr (I)	
	t/st (I)	
	d/ld (F)	
	g/gr (I)	
	d/ʤ (I)	
	t/ʧ (I)	

According to this test's norms, /h/ is mastered by 1½ years of age; /p/ is mastered by 2 years; /f/ and /k/ are mastered by 2½ years; and /j/ and /t/ are mastered by 3 years. The remaining errored phonemes are not expected to be mastered until 5 years or later. Therefore, according to the test norms, /f, k, j, p, t, h/ should have been mastered by Mary's age.

Mary's total score on this test was 71.5, which resulted in a standard score of 34 and a percentile of 6. This indicated a rating of "moderate" severity. Mary's intelligibility score was ranked level 4, which is interpreted as "speech is intelligible with careful listening."

Stimulability was performed to determine whether Mary could imitate errored phonemes when given an auditory model. She was stimulable for /h/, /f/, and /j/ in the initial position of words. She was not stimulable for the remainder of the errored phonemes.

continues

Exhibit 4–1 continued

A sample of Mary's conversational speech was obtained to compare articulation on single words with articulation in connected speech as well as to determine her intelligibility. It was found that the errors in connected speech were consistent with the errors on the formal test. Mary was unintelligible in 25% of her conversational speech.

Language Ability

Receptive

Mary's receptive language ability was not formally tested. Informal observation based on her ability to follow conversation and correctly answer questions indicated that her receptive language skills were within normal limits.

Expressive

Mary's expressive language ability was not formally assessed. Informal observation based on a sample of her conversation indicated that expressive language skills were within normal limits.

Oral Peripheral Examination

Structure

Mary's lips and tongue were of normal size, shape, and symmetry. The relationship of the mandible to the maxilla was normal. Examination of the hard and soft palate revealed no abnormalities.

Function

Mary was able to protrude, retract, elevate, depress, and lateralize her tongue. She was able to protrude and retract both her lips and her tongue in quick succession. Adequate velopharyngeal closure was evident on production of /ɑ/. Diadochokinetic rate was adequate as judged on production of /pʌtəkə/, even though articulatory errors were present on /t/ and /k/.

Vocal Parameters

Mary's vocal parameters were informally assessed during conversation. Her pitch, quality, and loudness were within normal limits for her age, gender, and size.

Auditory Sensitivity

An attempt was made to screen Mary's hearing by administering a pure-tone screening test. However, she could not be conditioned to raise her hand upon hearing a tone. Therefore, Mary's hearing was informally assessed. Because she responded to questions and conversation presented at varying intensity levels, her hearing is probably within normal limits. In addition, Mrs. Smith indicated that Mary had her hearing tested previously and she passed. Further details could not be obtained, as Mrs.

continues

Exhibit 4–1 continued

Smith could not remember where Mary was tested, who tested her, or when the testing had occurred.

Impressions

Mary exhibits an articulation problem of moderate severity that is characterized by omissions and substitutions. A reduction in intelligibility is evident. Careful listening is necessary to understand single words. In conversation, 75% of Mary's output can be understood. Prognosis for improvement with therapy is good, as Mary was stimulable to some of her errored phonemes.

Recommendations

It is recommended that:

1. Mary be enrolled in articulation therapy twice a week for individual half-hour sessions.
2. An attempt should be made to condition Mary so that reliable results can be obtained on a pure-tone hearing screening test.

Mary's initial therapeutic goals should be:

1. to produce /p, t, f, k/ correctly in the initial and final positions of words in sentences in 90% of her attempts
2. to produce /h/ correctly in the initial position of words in sentences in 90% of her attempts

Sally Doe
Sally Doe
Undergraduate Student Clinician

Betty A. Brown, M.S. CCC/SLP
Betty A. Brown, M.S. CCC/SLP
Clinical Supervisor

Exhibit 4–2 Sample Evaluation

[Identifying Information]

NAME:	Carlos R.	FILE NUMBER:	
ADDRESS:	00 Mill Road	EVALUATION DATE:	October 17, [this year]
	Maintown, PA 00000	BIRTHDATE:	March 1, [4 years ago]
PHONE:	000-000-0000	AGE:	3 years, 8 months
PARENTS:	Carlos and Sally	CLINICIAN:	Mary Miller
PROBLEM:	Language	SEMESTER:	Fall [this year]

SPEECH-LANGUAGE EVALUATION

Background Information

Carlos R., age 3 years, 8 months, was initially screened for speech and language problems at the Middletown Head Start Center on September 26 of this year. The service was provided by a student from the Speech and Hearing Center, Maintown University. At that time, the **Fluharty Preschool Speech and Language Screening Test** was administered. Carlos' chronological age at that time was 3 years, 7 months. The results were as follows:

Identification Total = 5	Cut-off Score = 11
Articulation Total = 26	Cut-off Score = 19
Comprehension Total = 6	Cut-off Score = 6
Repetition Total = 2	Cut-off Score = 4

Carlos passed the articulation and comprehension portions of the test but failed the identification and repetition sections. Therefore, further evaluation was warranted. Thus, Carlos was seen for a language evaluation on October 17.

An informant was not present. Therefore, background information had to be obtained from Carlos' file at his Head Start Center. According to the file, Carlos' medical history was not characterized by any illnesses or hospitalizations. It was also documented in the files that Carlos met his childhood milestones for motoric skills and normal speech and language development at the appropriate ages. However, specific ages were not available for when each milestone was met.

Spanish is Carlos' native language and is the primary language spoken in his home. However, Carlos' mother speaks English fluently. Mrs. R.'s description of Carlos, which appeared in his file, was "hyperactive." It was also noted in the file that Carlos' parents were separated since he was 1 year, 6 months of age. Carlos lives with his mother and three brothers. It was also reported in the file that Carlos' father visits regularly.

continues

Exhibit 4–2 continued

Additional information can be found in Carlos' file located at his Head Start Center.

Evaluation

Carlos was cooperative during testing. He attempted all tasks.

Language Ability

Receptive

The **Peabody Picture Vocabulary Test-Revised** (Form M) was administered to assess Carlos' performance on receptive vocabulary. His raw score of 8 resulted in a standard score equivalent of 61, a percentile rank less than 1, a stanine score of 1, and an age equivalent of 2 years, 2 months. His performance was 1 year, 6 months below his chronological age.

Carlos correctly identified the following vocabulary words: "car," "ball," "money," "bee," "bottle," "circle," "plant," and "ladder." He did not correctly identify the following: "broom," "candle," "reading," "full," "mail," "horn," and "pulling."

Carlos' receptive language was informally assessed. He responded appropriately to all questions asked and followed commands without difficulty. He was able to perform the following upon request: go to a shelf and select a specific toy, make a toy horse walk and jump, show how a toy worked, and put various animals in the barn.

Expressive

The **Expressive One-Word Picture Vocabulary Test** was administered to assess Carlos' expressive semantic skills. His raw score of 27 resulted in a mental age of 2 years, 9 months, a percentile of 3, and a stanine score of 2. His raw score was 1.3 standard deviations below the median. His performance was 11 months below his chronological age. He was able to name the following: "boat," "cat," "apple," "eyes," "bus," "tree," "bear," "truck," "train," "glasses," "duck," "knife," "hammer," "scissors," "chicken," and "tiger." Carlos did not name the following: "pumpkin" (no response), "umbrella" (response was "rain"), "wagon" (response was "bus"), "kite" (response was "balloon"), "triangle" (response was "star"), "square" (response was "circle"), "ear" (response was "nose"), "wheel" (response was "boat"), "leaf" (response was "tree"), and "typewriter" (response was "Go like this" as typing movements were demonstrated).

The **Structured Photographic Expressive Language Test-Preschool** was administered to assess expressive language skills. Carlos' raw score of 2 placed him below the first percentile. He scored 5 standard deviations below the mean. Errors were noted on the following structures: prepositions, plural nouns /s/, /z/, and /ɪz/, plural present progressive tense verbs, possessive nouns, subject pronouns, singular

continues

Exhibit 4–2 continued

present progressive tense verbs, regular past tense verbs, third-person singular copula "is," third-person plural copula "are," third-person singular marker on present tense of the verb, simple negation, and irregular past tense verbs. Better than 80% of the children in Carlos' age group (3–6 to 3–11) had success on these structures. Structures on which less than 80% of the children had success were third-person singular, regular past tense, simple negation, and irregular past tense. Therefore, Carlos did not demonstrate age-appropriate syntactic skills.

An informal language sample was obtained to assess expressive language skills in spontaneous conversation. A mean length of utterance was computed from the sample. It was 4.14 with an upper bound of 11. According to Brown's stages, Carlos is functioning in Stage 5. Some examples of his utterances are "I wanna check one more time," "Right here there are two turtles," "What do you got there?" "What is that?" "Is it like that?" "I wanna put that back," "It could fall down on the book," "But this will take it off," "This don't fit right there," "The Ninja Turtle can't fit," "I have those at home," "I'm gonna put the cow right here," "It came out," "It broke the window," "It's running," and "I will get it."

Oral Peripheral Examination

Structure

Carlos' lips and tongue were of normal size, shape, and symmetry. The relationship of the mandible to the maxilla was within normal limits. The soft palate appeared to be within normal limits. However, the hard palate was extremely high and narrow.

Function

Carlos was able to protrude and retract his lips. He could also perform these movements in quick succession. Carlos could elevate, depress, protrude, retract, and lateralize his tongue. Velopharyngeal closure was assessed on production of /ɑ/ and found to be within normal limits. Diadochokinetic rate was not within normal limits as productions were slow and arrhythmic.

Vocal Parameters

Pitch and loudness were within normal limits for Carlos' age, gender, and size. Vocal quality was slightly hyponasal. However, Carlos appeared to have a cold, as there were several episodes of sneezing and coughing throughout the evaluation.

Auditory Sensitivity

A pure-tone hearing screening test was administered to assess Carlos' hearing sensitivity. The frequencies 500, 1000, 2000, and 4000 were tested at 25 dB. Carlos responded correctly to all frequencies in both ears.

continues

Exhibit 4–2 continued

Impressions

Formal test results indicate that Carlos' receptive and expressive language skills are not commensurate with his chronological age. However, informal assessment of his receptive and expressive language reveals very different results in that Carlos' language functioning was appropriate for his chronological age. In Carlos' case, it is believed that formal test results are not a true indication of his language functioning.

Recommendations

Language therapy is not warranted at this time, as informal assessment indicated functioning within normal limits. However, owing to the disparity found between formal and informal results, Carlos' language should be re-evaluated during the forthcoming spring semester.

Mary Miller
_____

Mary Miller
Undergraduate Student Clinician

Betty A. Brown, M.S. CCC/SLP
_____

Betty A. Brown, M.S. CCC/SLP
Clinical Supervisor

Exhibit 4–3 Sample Evaluation

[Identifying Information]

NAME:	Patrick A.	FILE NUMBER:	
ADDRESS:	00 Main Street	EVALUATION DATE:	June 30, [this year]
	Maintown	BIRTHDATE:	June 00, [5 years ago]
	PA 00000	AGE:	5 years, 0 months
PHONE:	000-0000	CLINICIAN:	Jane Smith
PARENTS:	Mary and John	SEMESTER:	Fall [last year]
PROBLEM:	Language and		
	Articulation		

SPEECH-LANGUAGE EVALUATION

Background Information

Patrick A., a Caucasian male age 5 years, 0 months, was seen at the Maintown University Speech and Hearing Clinic on June 30 of this year. He was referred by Mary Jones, a speech-language pathologist, at Maintown Hospital's Speech and Hearing Center. Patrick's father, Mr. A., accompanied him to the evaluation and served as the informant during the case history interview.

Regarding prenatal history, it was reported that Mrs. A. was under a physician's care throughout her pregnancy. Mr. A. reported that the pregnancy was "normal" with no illness, emotional upset, or special diet. Concerning natal history, Mrs. A.'s labor lasted approximately 7 hours and Patrick was born by cesarean section. According to the informant, Patrick's birth weight was 7 pounds, 3 ounces. Postnatal history revealed that Patrick has had all immunizations to date and has not had any childhood diseases. It was also reported that when Patrick was approximately 2½ to 3 years of age, he was hospitalized for 2 weeks due to urinal retention. When asked to describe Patrick's general health, Mr. A. reported that it was "good."

According to the informant, there were no speech or language problems in the family. It was reported by Mr. A. that he himself has a slight hearing loss. When asked to compare Patrick's development to that of other children, Mr. A. stated, "his physical development is normal. He is below others in social/emotional development and language or communication skills."

Patrick's motor development was described as "normal." However, Mr. A. stated that Patrick is still in the process of toilet training. It was reported that Patrick is able to dress himself but still has difficulty with snaps and buttons. He is able to use crayons and pencils to draw and color.

---

continues

Exhibit 4–3 continued

With regard to social development, Mr. A. reported that Patrick's eye contact is not good but is presently improving. He also stated that Patrick enjoys playing with cars and looking at books when indoors. Outdoors, he enjoys playing on his swing set, riding his bike, and playing in his swimming pool. Mr. A. described Patrick's personality as "pleasant, but if he is frustrated, he can be nasty."

Concerning speech and language development, Mr. A. reported that Patrick babbled and his first word, "dada," appeared around 15 months. It was also reported that Patrick started putting words together at 2½ to 3 years of age. Mr. A. reported that at the present time, Patrick speaks in short phrases or is echolalic. His vocabulary was reported to consist of several hundred words. Mr. A. also stated that Patrick occasionally uses gestures alone or in combination with short phrases. Patrick's speech/language problem was first noticed when he was around 18 months to 2 years of age.

Information regarding education was obtained. Patrick is currently attending the Head Start program. Mr. A. stated that Patrick gets along well with his teachers and peers. Reportedly, Patrick receives speech and language therapy once a week for 30 minutes.

In addition, Mr. A. reported that "a few months ago," Patrick went through a period of "speaking with a rough voice." He also reported that at this time the "roughness" has disappeared.

Evaluation

Patrick was initially unwilling to separate from his father. He sat on his father's lap for a few minutes while refusing to cooperate. However, he showed interest in the testing materials and was easily enticed into cooperating. Once Patrick became involved in the testing procedure, Mr. A. was able to leave the room. It was sometimes difficult to keep Patrick on task during testing. Token reinforcement was necessary during part of the evaluation in order to maintain Patrick's attention. Periodically during the evaluation, Patrick turned away and started whining when he did not want to continue. This behavior appeared to increase as the test items became more difficult.

General Language

The **Mecham Verbal Language Development Scale**, a parent report inventory that assesses a child's general language ability, was administered to Mr. A. A language age equivalent of 4 years, 6½ months was obtained.

Receptive Language

The **Peabody Picture Vocabulary Test**, form L, was administered to assess single word receptive vocabulary skill through picture identification. However, a basal of

continues

Exhibit 4–3 continued

eight consecutive correct responses could not be obtained. Therefore, an estimate of Patrick's receptive vocabulary could not be made.

The **Preschool Language Scale-3 (PLS-3)** was administered to assess Patrick's ability to receive auditory information involving concrete and abstract concepts, parts of speech, and grammatical language features. Patrick's raw score of 34 corresponds to an Auditory Comprehension Age of 3 years, 5 months. Weaknesses noted included recognizing actions, distinguishing parts, grouping objects, distinguishing prepositions, and understanding the concept of "three." Strengths were not evident.

Expressive Language

The expressive communication portion of the **PLS-3** was administered to measure vocabulary, verbalized memory span, concrete and abstract thought, concept acquisition, articulation, and the ability to use grammatical features of language. A raw score of 26 was obtained, which corresponds to an Expressive Communication Age of 2 years, 10 months. Weaknesses noted included using pronouns, naming objects, using plurals, conversing in sentences, answering questions logically, repeating sentences, stating opposites, and telling about remote events. Areas of strength were not evident.

During the evaluation, Patrick often imitated the clinician's utterances and intonation patterns. The function of these echoic responses was to maintain communication.

A 10-minute sample of Patrick's communication with the clinician during play was recorded. Interactions, intents, and consequences of the communication sample were analyzed to obtain pragmatic information. Patrick's interactions were classified as initiating, responding, or maintaining behaviors through the three modes of paralinguistic, vocal, and verbal. His role in the interaction can be classified as follows:

	Paralinguistic	*Vocal*	*Verbal*	*Total*
Initiating	$0/86 = 0\%$	$5/86 = 6\%$	$6/86 = 7\%$	$11/86 = 13\%$
Responding	$2/86 = 2\%$	$14/86 = 16\%$	$29/86 = 34\%$	$45/86 = 52\%$
Maintaining	$0/86 = 0\%$	$10/86 = 12\%$	$19/86 = 22\%$	$29/86 = 34\%$

Included in the vocal category were nine quick, short ventricular phonations that Patrick produced spontaneously. These included two instances of initiating, three of maintaining, and four responding behaviors during the 10-minute sample. These voiced gasps were often produced in conjunction with other communication behaviors (e.g., pointing) during the entire evaluation.

In addition, 42 spontaneous, intelligible verbal communicative behaviors were analyzed according to communicative intent by categorizing them as instrumentals $(22/42 = 52\%)$, statements $(20/42 = 48\%)$, or negations $(0/42 = 0\%)$. The instrumentals and statements were categorized as follows:

continues

Exhibit 4–3 continued

Instrumentals		Statements	
Joint attention	3/42 = 7%	Informative	20/42 = 48%
Objects	3/42 = 7%	Emotive	0/42 = 0%
Actions	11/42 = 26%	Social	0/42 = 0%
Regulation of behavior	5/42 = 12%	Experimental	0/42 = 0%
Assistance	0/42 = 0%		
Information	0/42 = 0%		

Negative behaviors indicating rejection, nonexistence, or denial were not evident in the sample.

A semantic case analysis was performed on the 42 intelligible, nonechoic responses. Little semantic diversity was evident; however, the following semantic relations were observed: (Note: Only semantic relations used two or more times are listed.)

Action + Locative (e.g., "Put in the box")	14/42 = 33%
Action + Object (e.g., "Open the door")	4/42 = 10%
Experiencer + State + Entity (e.g., "I want baby")	2/42 = 5%
Action + Object + Locative (e.g., "Put it in the chair")	2/42 = 5%

A Type Token Ratio was computed on the 42 intelligible, nonechoic utterances to explore Patrick's use of referential meaning. The total number of different words Patrick produced was divided by the total number of words produced. A Type Token Ratio of 0.29 (32/110) was obtained, which indicates that there was very little lexical diversity evident in the sample.

The mean length of utterance (MLU) was determined from the utterances in the 10-minute language sample. The MLU was calculated to be 3.17 morphemes when echoic utterances were excluded. The mean length of all verbal utterances was calculated to be 3.02 morphemes, which corresponds to a predicted chronological age of 34.8 months with a standard deviation of 6.8 months. Patrick's chronological age of 58 months places him 3 standard deviations below the mean. This MLU corresponds to Brown's Stage IV. Structures normally evident at this stage that were not observed in Patrick's sample include correct use of auxiliary verbs, copulas, prepositions "on," "with," "of," "for," and "to," demonstrative pronouns "this" and "that," personal pronouns "you," "me," and "my," and plural noun inflections /s/, /z/, and /ɪz/.

Speech

The **Goldman-Fristoe Test of Articulation** was administered to assess single-word articulation skills. When spontaneous productions could not be obtained, productions were obtained imitatively. Forty-nine errors were recorded of a total of 73 phonemes tested for in an inaccuracy of 67%. The following errors were noted:

continues

Exhibit 4–3 continued

	Initial	*Medial*	*Final*	*Blends*	
p	*	—	*	bl	b/bl
m		X*	—	br	b/br
n	X			dr	w/dr
b		*	*	fl	f/fl
g	k/g		ʔ/g	kl	kw/kl*
k		ʔ/k	—	kr	b/kr
f	*			pl	ʔ/pl
d	*			skw	θkw/skw*
ŋ		ʔ/ŋ		sl	θ/sl
j	1/j			st	θ/st
ʃ	s/ʃ*	X*	X*	tr	tw/tr
ʧ	t/ʧ*	t/ʧ*	θ/ʧ*	hw	w/hw*
r	w/r	w/r	—		
ʤ	d/ʤ*	d/ʤ*			
θ	f/θ	f/θ			
v	b/v	f/v			
s	d/s*	X*	X*		
z	d/z				
ð	d/ð*	d/ð			

Key: ʔ = glottal stop; X = distortion; — = omission; * = interdental or labiodental.

Although some sounds were judged as correct perceptually, they were produced with incorrect placement. Many phonemes were produced with either interdental or labiodental placement. Informal analysis revealed that the following phonological processes were evident: final consonant deletion (/dʌ/ for /drʌm/ and /dʌ/ for /dʌk/), devoicing (/kʌn/ for /gʌn/), and stopping (d/s, d/z, and d/ð). Patrick was stimulable for /p, m, n, k/ at the syllable, word, and two-word phrase level. He was also able to imitate /d/ at all levels, although it was made labiodentally. Patrick was stimulable for /j/ at the syllable and word levels. Imitatively. Patrick's intelligibility is good, although the intelligibility of his spontaneous speech is poor.

Voice

The vocal parameters were informally assessed during conversation. Pitch and loudness were within normal limits for Patrick's age, gender, and size. However, his quality varied from breathy to normal to strained. Ventricular phonations were also produced in the manner of voiced gasps.

Auditory Sensitivity

An attempt was made to administer a pure-tone hearing screening test. Results could not be obtained because Patrick would not wear the headset. However, he did

continues

Exhibit 4–3 continued

not have any difficulty hearing speech at varying levels of loudness throughout the evaluation.

Oral Peripheral Examination

Structure

Patrick's lips and tongue were of normal size, shape, and symmetry. The relationship of the mandible to the maxilla was within normal limits. Examination of the hard and soft palate revealed no abnormalities.

Function

Patrick rounded his lips, placed his upper teeth on his lower lip, elevated, depressed, and lateralized his tongue tip upon imitation. Velopharyngeal closure was adequate on production of /ɑ/. Patrick's diadochokinetic rate was within normal limits on production of /pʌtəkə/.

Impressions

Patrick exhibits a moderate delay in receptive language, a moderate to severe delay in expressive language, and a moderate delay in articulation. Prognosis for improvement is favorable. Positive prognostic indicators include stimulability for errored phonemes as well as his young age. A negative prognostic sign is that an impairment exists in all areas tested—receptive language, expressive language, and articulation.

Recommendations

It is recommended that Patrick continue to receive speech and language therapy. If possible, he should be seen three times a week. A low structured setting centering around Patrick's interests and daily routines may be beneficial. Relevant linguistic codes provided by the speech-language pathologist within this setting may stimulate similar relevant verbalizations from Patrick. Modification of Patrick's environment by creating various contextual situations may enhance his ability to induce content–form–use interactions. By providing appropriate contexts and functions, Patrick's attempts to use content/form interactions will be promptly rewarded by his successful communication. Modeling successful communication by another child may also be beneficial. In this manner, Patrick can first observe another child's effective use of appropriate form/content behaviors. Interpersonal functions of language (commenting about ongoing events, pretend or fantasy, and expression of emotion) can also be incorporated into the intervention procedures.

The following receptive language goals are recommended:

1. to increase recognition of actions
2. to improve ability to distinguish parts

continues

Exhibit 4–3 continued

3. to improve ability to categorize objects
4. to increase receptive vocabulary
5. to improve ability to distinguish prepositions

The following expressive language goals are recommended:

1. to increase the number of utterances that serve interpersonal functions (e.g., to obtain objects—"I want baby"; to regulate behavior of others—"Sit down"; and to call attention to self or objects and events in the environment—"Look")
2. to produce utterances in order to obtain information or assistance ("Help me")
3. to increase the number of utterances that are initiated by Patrick through joint attention activities (identify objects or events that Patrick takes an interest in—"Baby." Promptly reinforce all of Patrick's attempts at initiation.)
4. to eliminate inappropriate echoic responses
5. to eliminate inappropriate vocal behaviors
6. to increase semantic diversity by coding Agent + Action, Agent + Object, Agent + Action + Object, and Agent + Action + Object + Place relations
7. to produce pronoun + noun combinations in coding possession
8. to increase correct use of auxiliary verbs, copulas, prepositions, and plural nouns

The following articulation goal is recommended:

1. to produce /p, m, k, g, ŋ, ʃ, ʧ/ correctly in spontaneous speech

Jane Smith
_____

Jane Smith
Undergraduate Student Clinician

Betty A. Brown, M.S. CCC/SLP
_____

Betty A. Brown, M.S. CCC/SLP
Clinical Supervisor

Exhibit 4–4 Sample Evaluation

Identifying Information

NAME: William Smith   FILE NUMBER:
ADDRESS: 00 Maintown Lane EVALUATION DATE: September 9 [this year]
              Maintown,   BIRTHDATE: March 14, [20 years ago]
              PA 00000   AGE: 20 years
PHONE: 000-000-0000   CLINICIAN: Jane Doe
PROBLEM: Fluency   SEMESTER: Fall [this year]

FLUENCY EVALUATION

Background Information

William Smith, age 20, presently attends Maintown University. His major is unde-clared at this time. His speech was evaluated at Maintown University's Speech and Hearing Center on September 9 of this year.

William's speech problem was diagnosed in fourth grade as stuttering. Fluency therapy was received for 8 years in public school. He also received therapy from Easter Seals. William indicated that these two therapy programs, which he received simultaneously, were not coordinated and contradicted each other. However, he was not able to provide details about the therapy received while enrolled in either pro-gram. William stated that his fluency problem has worsened over the years. He is very aware of his problem and would very much like to remediate it.

On the case history form, William indicated that his stuttering becomes more se-vere when he is in a new situation. He also indicated that his stuttering worsens when he is under stress. When around familiar people, William does not have as much difficulty. He indicated that he has no history of hearing problems, respiratory prob-lems, or any illnesses or accidents that could have caused his speech problem.

Evaluation

William was very attentive during this evaluation. He was extremely cooperative. All tasks were performed completely and willingly.

Fluency

The **Fluency Interview** was administered to assess the number of stuttered words William had in various contexts. The results were:

continues

Exhibit 4–4 continued

Task	*Part-Word*	*Struggle*	*Prolongation*	*Time*
		Type of Stuttering		
Automatic		1		44 sec.
Echoic		2	3	14 sec.
Reading	6	4		54 sec.
Pictures		1		3 sec.
Monologue	2	1		47 sec.
Questions	1	2	1	20 sec.
Conversation	1	2	1	39 sec.
Observation in another setting	11	2		42 sec.

Overall total = 4 minutes 23 seconds or 4.38 minutes

Part-word repetitions = 21
Struggles = 15
Prolongations = 5

Total Stuttered Words/Minute = 9.36

According to the **Fluency Interview** norms, a normal speaker should not exceed a rate of 0.5 stuttered words per minute. William's rate exceeds this limit by 8.86 stuttered words per minute.

The *Stuttering Severity Instrument (SSI)* was administered to assess William's fluency during reading and conversation. The results were:

Frequency Task Score = 12
Duration Score = 4
Total Physical Concomitant Score = 9
Total Overall Score = 25
Severity = Moderate

According to the **SSI** test norms, William is exhibiting stuttering of moderate severity. The estimated length of his three longest blocks was approximately 3 seconds. He exhibited all four of the physical concomitants: distracting sounds (score, 2); facial grimaces (score, 3); head movements (score, 3); and movement of extremities (score, 1).

Auditory Sensitivity

A pure-tone hearing screening test was administered to ascertain whether hearing was within normal limits. William responded to 25 dB tones in his right and left ears at all frequencies presented (250, 500, 1000, 2000, and 4000 Hz).

continues

Exhibit 4–4 continued

Oral Peripheral Examination

Structure

The structure of the oral mechanism is adequate for normal speech production.

Function

The function of William's oral mechanism is adequate for normal speech production.

Vocal Parameters

Pitch, quality, and loudness are within normal limits for William's age, gender, and size.

Impressions

William has a stuttering problem of moderate severity. Because of his awareness of his problem and strong desire to change it, prognosis for improvement is good.

Recommendations

It is recommended that William be enrolled immediately to receive fluency therapy. He should be seen individually for two half-hour sessions per week. The following goals should be emphasized:

1. to stutter fewer than 0.5 stuttered words per minute during reading
2. to stutter fewer than 0.5 stuttered words per minute during monologue
3. to stutter fewer than 0.5 stuttered words per minute during conversation

Jane Smith
_____
Jane Smith
Undergraduate Student Clinician

Betty A. Brown, M.S. CCC/SLP
_____
Betty A. Brown, M.S. CCC/SLP
Clinical Supervisor

is evident in any area of speech or language, it should be addressed. The structure and function of the oral peripheral mechanism do not need to be written in detail as long as problems are not evident. Likewise, it is not necessary to discuss vocal parameters in any detail. If, however, a problem is evident in any of these areas, it should be addressed thoroughly.

QUICK CHECK

Take the time to read and reread your evaluations upon completion. Make certain they "shine." If they do not, determine the problematic area(s) and rewrite.

RE-EVALUATIONS—SAMPLES

Differences between an evaluation and a re-evaluation can be seen most vividly in the background information section. A re-evaluation will not include all the information contained in the initial evaluation, but it will refer the reader to the previous evaluation by date or to the client's entire file. Previous therapy may be cited in this section. Additional differences might be seen in the oral peripheral examination and hearing sensitivity sections. In most cases, if these areas were within normal limits when previously evaluated, they will not be evaluated again.

Re-Evaluation One: Articulation and Language

This re-evaluation (Exhibit 4–5) focuses on articulation as well as receptive and expressive language. This child's native language is Spanish.

Re-Evaluation Two: Voice

The focus of this re-evaluation (Exhibit 4–6) is voice. Therefore, aspects pertinent to voice will be emphasized. It is important for you to have some additional information. Before receiving therapy, this client was referred to an otolaryngologist in order to obtain the status of the vocal cords. This previous report can be found in her file. The results of this evaluation revealed a "normal" larynx.

QUICK CHECK

When you are done writing your re-evaluations, reread them. Make certain they are reports of which you are proud.

Exhibit 4–5 Sample Re-Evaluation

[Identifying Information]

NAME: Vicente M.   FILE NUMBER:
ADDRESS: 00 Main Lane   DATE: March 10, [this year]
         Maintown, PA 00000   BIRTHDATE: October 4, [5 years ago]
PHONE: 000-000-0000   AGE: 4 years, 5 months
PARENT: S.   CLINICIAN: Mary Doe
PROBLEM: Articulation and Language SEMESTER: Spring [this year]

Background Information

    Vicente M. is 4 years, 5 months old. He attends the afternoon nursery class at the Maintown Nursery Center. He has been receiving services from Maintown University's Speech and Hearing Center since the fall of last year. These services were provided by a student clinician. Because Vicente was evaluated in November of the fall semester, he was placed in group language stimulation where the emphasis was placed on naming body parts in English. Vicente's native language is Spanish, and this is the language spoken in his home. His English vocabulary is quite limited. Please refer to his initial evaluation dated November 10 of last year for further information.

Evaluation

    Vicente was very quiet. It was difficult for him to attend to a task for more than 10 minutes.

Speech

    The **Goldman-Fristoe Test of Articulation** was administered to assess Vicente's articulation on single words. The results were:

Substitutions		*Omissions*	
Consonants	*Blends*	*Consonants*	*Blends*
v/b (M)	kw/kl	/m/ (M)	/r/ in /dr/
s/f (F)	pw/pl	/n/ (F)	/l/ in /fl/
t/d (F)	sk/skw	/b/ (F)	

continues

Exhibit 4–5 continued

Consonants	Blends	Consonants	Blends
t/ʃ (F)	tw/tr	/g/ (F)	
t/ʧ (I)		/ŋ/ (F)	
ʃ /ʧ (M,F)		/v/ (F)	
w/l (F)		/z/ (F)	
w/r (M,F)			
j/ʤ (F)			
ʃ/ʤ (F)			
f/θ (I)			
d/θ (M,F)			
b/v (I,M)			
d/z (M)			
d/ð (I,M)			

According to Sander's norms, the phonemes /m/, /n/, and /b/ should be mastered before age 2 and /g/, /ŋ/, and /d/ should be mastered at age 2. The phonemes /f/, /r/, and /l/ should be mastered at 3 years of age. At 4 years of age, the phonemes /ʧ/, /ʃ/, /ʤ/, /z/, and /v/ should be mastered. Because Vicente is 4 years, 5 months, the phonemes just listed should all be mastered. Vicente's other errored phonemes are not expected to be mastered at his age. However, many of his misarticulations may be the result of his Spanish-speaking background. Vicente had 34 errors, which resulted in a percentile rank of 4.

Vicente's stimulability was assessed to determine which errored phonemes could be imitated in the initial, medial, and final positions of syllables, words, and sentences. It was found that Vicente was stimulable on /v/ in the initial, medial, and final position of words in sentences; /n/ in the initial and medial position of words in sentences; /ʃ/, /l/, and /d/ in the initial, medial, and final position of words; /f/ in the initial and final position of words; and /b/ in the initial and medial position of words. Vicente was not stimulable for other errored phonemes at any level.

A conversational speech sample was taken to determine intelligibility, to assess ability to articulate in connected speech, and to compare misarticulations in conversation to misarticulations on the **Goldman-Fristoe Test of Articulation**. The results indicated that Vicente is unintelligible in connected speech when the context is not known. When context is known, only a few key words are intelligible. Errors noted in conversation were consistent with errors noted on the formal articulation test.

Language

Receptive

The **Preschool Language Scale-3 (PLS-3)** was administered to assess receptive language formally. Vicente's raw score of 28 resulted in a standard score of 70, a

continues

Exhibit 4–5 continued

percentile rank of 2, and an age equivalent of 2 years, 10 months. Performance is 17 months below his chronological age. Vicente passed all items between the ages of 2–6 and 2–11 that included descriptive concepts, part and whole relationships, and understanding pronouns. However, he did not perform successfully on items between the ages of 3–0 and 3–11 that included understanding negatives, comparing objects, or indicating body parts on himself.

Expressive

The **Preschool Language Scale-3 (PLS-3)** was administered to assess expressive language formally. Vicente's raw score of 20 is equivalent to a standard score of 61, a percentile rank of 0, and an age equivalent of 2 years, 2 months. His performance is 2 years, 3 months below his chronological age. Vicente passed all items between the ages of 1–6 and 1–11 that included having a vocabulary of at least 10 words, naming objects, producing a succession of single-word utterances, and using one pronoun. Vicente was not successful on the next age level (2–0 to 2–11), as he was not able to combine three or four words in spontaneous speech, answer Wh questions, produce basic sentences, or use possessives.

A language sample was obtained to further assess expressive language. The majority of Vicente's responses consisted of single words used for labeling. Expanded utterances could not be elicited. However, Vicente asked one question, which was "What's that?" Twenty-five utterances, containing 32 morphemes, were obtained, which resulted in a mean length of utterance of 1.3. This placed Vicente in Brown's first stage of early language development. These results were consistent with formal testing.

Overall Language

Vicente's standard score total of his receptive and expressive performance was 131, which resulted in a total language standard score of 62, a percentile rank of 1, and an age equivalent of 2 years, 7 months. He is functioning 1 year 10 months below his chronological age.

Oral Peripheral Examination

Structure

Vicente's lips and tongue were of normal size, shape, and symmetry. The relationship of the mandible to the maxilla was within normal limits. Examination of the hard and soft palate revealed no abnormalities.

Function

Vicente rounded his lips, placed his upper teeth on his lower lip, elevated, depressed, and lateralized his tongue tip. Velopharyngeal closure was adequate on production of /ɑ/. Diadochokinetic rate was within normal limits as assessed on production of /pʌtəkə/.

continues

Exhibit 4–5 continued

Auditory Sensitivity

A pure-tone hearing screening test was not administered as hearing sensitivity was within normal limits when previously assessed on November 10 last year. Informal assessment during this re-evaluation further indicated that hearing was not a problem at this time.

Impressions

Vicente has a severe receptive and severe expressive language impairment in English, which is probably the result of Spanish being his native language, as well as Spanish being the only language spoken in his home. Vicente also has a severe articulation problem in English. However, a number of his misarticulations are the result of his Spanish-speaking background. It is thought that with continual language stimulation in English, Vicente's ability to imitate words will improve, and if Vicente's attention can be maintained, prognosis for improvement of the English language is favorable.

Recommendations

It is recommended that Vicente receive language therapy on an individual basis three times a week for half-hour sessions. It is further recommended that Vicente's receptive and expressive Spanish be evaluated to make certain that an impairment exists only in English. Goals should consist of:

1. correct receptive identification of pictures in 90% of his attempts
2. correct expressive identification of pictures in 90% of his attempts
3. correct categorization of pictures in 90% of his attempts

Jane Smith
_____
Jane Smith
Undergraduate Student Clinician

Betty A. Brown, M.S. CCC/SLP
_____
Betty A. Brown, M.S. CCC/SLP
Clinical Supervisor

Exhibit 4–6 Sample Re-Evaluation

[Identifying Information]

NAME: Alice K.   FILE NUMBER:
ADDRESS: 001 Main Street   EVALUATION DATE: October 8 [this year]
             Maintown, PA 00000   BIRTHDATE: May 2 [21 years ago]
PHONE: 000-000-0000   AGE: 21 years
PROBLEM: Voice   CLINICIAN: Mary Jones
                                                     SEMESTER: Fall [this year]

Background Information

Alice K. is 21 years old. She received voice therapy during the spring semester last year at Maintown University's Speech and Hearing Center. Therapy focused on the use of relaxation techniques in order to improve vocal quality. Progress was made throughout the semester, although occasional regression was noted. Alice's long-term goal of using good vocal quality during conversation in 90% of her attempts was not met. A re-evaluation took place on September 22 of this year.

Alice described definite vocal abuse situations. She also stated that her voice tires after using it for an extended amount of time. Please refer to her file for additional information.

Evaluation

Vocal Parameters

The **Voice Assessment Protocol for Children and Ad**   was administered to assess Alice's pitch, loudness, and quality. Breathing, as well as rate of speech, was also assessed.

Pitch

Alice's habitual pitch was 196 Hz, which corresponds with the musical note G3. This was found by having her count to 5 and prolong the vowels. Her optimal pitch was 293 Hz, which corresponds with the musical note D4. This was determined by using both the Loud-Sigh Technique and the natural speech method. Alice's pitch ranges from 169 Hz to 659 Hz. In musical terms, Alice's range goes from C3 to E5. It was observed that Alice did not use her optimal pitch while speaking. Instead she used a lower pitch. This lower-pitched voice seemed to be a habit. Pitch breaks were not demonstrated, and normal inflections were used.

Loudness

Alice demonstrated a typical level of loudness that was comfortably maintained. Her range of loudness was normal and was evenly emphasized. She has specific situ-

continues

Exhibit 4–6 continued

ations in her life, such as band and teaching twirling, that cause her to use increased loudness levels.

Quality

The quality of Alice's voice was assessed. Her voice was moderately breathy and hoarse. There was a definite harsh strain heard in her voice. Her speech was also characterized by slight hypernasality.

Breath Features

Speech breathing was assessed. Alice used the clavicular region. A slight audible inhalation was evident during speech breathing. Alice stated that she uses an excessive amount of words per breath. She also commented that she sometimes runs out of breath when trying to finish sentences. Alice was able to prolong the /ɑ/ sound for the normal amount of time, but her voice fatigued toward the end. The s/z ratio was 1.07, which suggested a normal larynx, but her voice tired at the end.

Rate

Alice's rate of speech was assessed. Her rate of 180 words per minute was within normal limits.

Connected Speech

A sample of conversation was obtained to assess Alice's voice in connected speech, compare findings to those obtained during formal testing, and evaluate intelligibility. Alice's voice was found to be breathy and harsh with slight hypernasality. Her breathing was clavicular instead of diaphragmatic. Alice's speech was intelligible. The problems found in connected speech were consistent with those found during formal testing.

Oral Peripheral Examination

An oral peripheral examination was performed to assess the structure and functioning of the oral mechanism.

Structure

Alice's oral structures are adequate for speech production.

Function

Alice had some difficulty performing diadochokinetic movements. While repeating /p/, /t/, and /k/ individually in rapid succession and while repeating /pʌtəkə/, her voice demonstrated fatigue.

continues

Exhibit 4–6 continued

Auditory Sensitivity

No formal hearing test was administered at this time. Alice's hearing was found to be within normal limits when tested last semester. Based on informal assessment, there was no reason to question whether her hearing status changed.

Impressions

According to the test results, Alice has a voice problem of moderate severity. Vocal quality is characterized as being breathy and hoarse with periodic episodes of a harsh strain. Both hypernasality and clavicular breathing are evident. With regard to pitch, Alice's habitual pitch is lower than her optimal pitch by 97 Hz. An improvement in quality would probably result in usage of optimal pitch. Alice frequently finds herself involved in vocal abuse situations. She is aware of these situations. Prognosis for improvement is good if Alice attends therapy and actively participates on a regular basis, applies facilitating techniques in all speaking situations, uses diaphragmatic breathing, and eliminates all episodes of vocal abuse.

Recommendations

It is recommended that Alice receive voice therapy twice a week on an individual basis. Sessions should be one-half hour in length. Goals should include:

1. using diaphragmatic breathing during conversation in 90% of her attempts
2. using good vocal quality during conversation in 90% of her attempts
3. decreasing the number of vocal abuse episodes to less than two per week

Jane Smith
_____

Jane Smith
Undergraduate Student Clinician

Betty A. Brown, M.S. CCC/SLP
_____

Betty A. Brown, M.S. CCC/SLP
Clinical Supervisor

PROGRESS REPORTS

A progress report is an after-the-fact report. It is a statement of a client's performance during therapy. The frequency with which a progress report is written varies pending the type of client as well as the setting. In a university setting, it is unfortunately the academic calendar that determines when such reports are written. Progress reports are usually written at the end of each semester. Exceptions may be made if the same clinician services a client for the entire university year (fall and spring semesters).

Progress Report One: Articulation

This progress report (Exhibit 4–7) indicates improvement in the area of articulation, but not enough to change the diagnosis. This client had difficulty self-monitoring; therefore, this aspect was not emphasized. Additional testing was not warranted.

Progress Report Two: Articulation

This progress report (Exhibit 4–8) also shows improvement in the area of articulation. Self-monitoring was emphasized. A comparison of formal test results is also included.

Progress Report Three: Language and Attending Behavior

Language and attending behavior are the areas of focus in this progress report (Exhibit 4–9). A comparison of formal test results is made.

QUICK CHECK

Check and recheck your progress reports. When progress is evident, make certain it is clearly stated. Make certain the procedures used to accomplish the various objectives are clear to the reader.

Exhibit 4–7 Sample Progress Report

[Identifying Information]

NAME: Mary Smith   FILE NUMBER:
ADDRESS: 00 Broad Street   DATE: April 30 [this year]
           Maintown, PA 00000   BIRTHDATE: December 9, [5 years ago]
PHONE: 000-000-0000   AGE: 4 years, 5 months
PARENTS: Mary and Bill   CLINICIAN: Sally Doe
PROBLEM: Articulation   SEMESTER: Spring [this year]

PROGRESS REPORT

Background Information

Mary Smith, age 4 years, 5 months, was seen for articulation therapy at the Speech and Hearing Center at Maintown University. She attended 20 sessions of the 23 held from February 6 to April 30 this year. Tests indicated that Mary's articulation errors consisted of the following substitutions: b/f, b/p, and g/k. Omissions of /h/ and /t/ were also evident. These errors resulted in unintelligibility at times. Please refer to previous reports for further information.

Therapeutic Objective

The long-range goal for this semester was to:

1. correctly produce /p, t, f, k/ in the initial, medial, and final positions of words in sentences and /h/ in the initial position of words in sentences during 90% of her attempts.

Progress and Procedures

Objective one (production of /p, t, f, k/ in all positions of words in sentences and /h/ in the initial position of words in sentences) was accomplished by first explaining how the articulators were used to produce speech sounds. Mary then imitated /p, t, f, k, h/ in isolation when given a model and a visual cue. Placement cues were given if necessary. When successful on imitation, Mary produced each phoneme after being shown a visual cue. She then progressed to imitating phonemes in CV [consonant–vowel] syllables, although branch steps were needed. The branch step for /p/ and /h/ consisted of production of the target sound followed by a pause and then the vowel sound. The branch step for /f/ consisted of prolonging /f/ and then producing the vowel sound. Mary imitated /p/, /t/, and /k/ in CV syllables and then progressed to production of VC [vowel–consonant] syllables. Imitation of /t, k, p/ in VC syllables was attempted next. A branch step of saying the vowel followed by a pause and then

continues

Exhibit 4–7 continued

saying /t/ was necessary. This step was accomplished by showing Mary the phoneme symbol card and modeling the syllable. Mary then advanced to a branch step that led her to the original objective of imitating the syllable without a branch step. She then progressed to the production of /p/, /t/, and /k/ in VC syllables. Mary then advanced to production of /k/ in words. She was shown pictures containing the target in the initial position and had to imitate a model.

Although the semester's goal was not met, progress was evident. Mary is now able to correctly imitate /p/ and /t/ in the initial position of syllables in 70% and 75% of her attempts, respectively. She is now able to produce /p/ and /t/ correctly in the final position of syllables in 100% and 90% of her attempts, respectively. The phonemes /f/ and /h/ are correctly imitated in the initial position of syllables in 90% and 85% of her attempts, respectively. The /k/ phoneme is correctly imitated in the initial position of words in 90% of her attempts.

Current Status and Impressions

Mary continues to exhibit an articulation problem of moderate severity that is characterized by omissions, substitutions, and a reduction in intelligibility. However, Mary is now able to correctly produce /p/ and /t/ in the final position of syllables, correctly imitate /f/ and /h/ in the initial position of syllables, and correctly imitate /k/ in the initial position of words. Based on Mary's good attendance, her active participation in therapy, Mrs. Smith's follow-through with all therapy assignments, and gains made thus far, prognosis for further improvement is favorable.

Recommendations

It is recommended that Mary be re-evaluated at the beginning of the forthcoming fall semester and continue to receive therapy if warranted. Possible goals for future therapy are:

1. to correctly produce /h, p, t, f/ in all positions of words in 90% of her attempts
2. to correctly produce /k/ in all positions of sentences in 90% of her attempts

Jane Smith
_____
Jane Smith
Undergraduate Student Clinician

Betty A. Brown, M.S. CCC/SLP
_____
Betty A. Brown, M.S. CCC/SLP
Clinical Supervisor

Exhibit 4–8 Sample Progress Report

[Identifying Information]

NAME: K. P.   FILE NUMBER:
ADDRESS: 01 Broad St.   DATE: May 14 [this year]
                 Maintown, PA 00000   BIRTHDATE: April 1 [19 years ago]
PHONE: 000-000-0000   AGE: 19
PROBLEM: Articulation   CLINICIAN: Sally Storm
                                                    SEMESTER: Spring [this year]

PROGRESS REPORT

Background Information

K. P., age 19, received therapy for a mild articulation problem from September 10 to December 12 during the fall semester last year. She was then re-evaluated at the Maintown University's Speech and Hearing Clinic on February 4 of this year. She continued to be diagnosed as having a mild articulation problem characterized by distortions of the /tʃ/ and /ʃ/ phonemes. Therefore, K. was again enrolled in therapy. This semester, the therapeutic emphasis was placed on correct production of the /ʃ/ phoneme in conversation. K. attended 26 of 28 sessions from February 4 to May 14. For further information, please refer to the client's file.

Therapeutic Objectives

The objectives for therapy were:

1. to enable K. to correctly produce the /ʃ/ phoneme as a releasor and arrestor in syllables in 90% of her attempts
2. to enable K. to correctly monitor her productions of the /ʃ/ phoneme as both releasor and arrestor in syllables in 90% of her attempts
3. to enable K. to correctly produce the /ʃ/ phoneme as a releasor and arrestor in words in 90% of her attempts
4. to enable K. to correctly monitor her productions of the /ʃ/ phoneme as both releasor and arrestor in words in 90% of her attempts
5. to enable K. to correctly produce the /ʃ/ phoneme as a releasor and arrestor in phrases in 90% of her attempts
6. to enable K. to correctly monitor her productions of the /ʃ/ phoneme as both releasor and arrestor in phrases in 90% of her attempts

continues

Exhibit 4–8 continued

7. to enable K. to correctly produce the /ʃ/ phoneme in conversation in 70% of her attempts
8. to enable K. to correctly monitor her productions of the /ʃ/ phoneme in conversation in 90% of her attempts

Progress and Procedures

Objective 1 (correct production of /ʃ/ in syllables) was accomplished by having K. correctly produce the /ʃ/ phoneme in isolation without a model. These productions were then incorporated into syllables as releasors and arrestors. K. was not able to correctly produce /ʃ/ in syllables at the beginning of the semester, but now produces it in 95% of her attempts.

Objective 2 (correct monitoring of /ʃ/ in syllables) was met by using ear training and tape recordings. K. was required to listen to recordings of her syllable lists and identify and self-correct each error. Her monitoring ability in syllables has increased from 10% at the beginning of the semester to 98% currently.

Objective 3 (production of /ʃ/ in words) was fulfilled by having K. incorporate her correct productions of the /ʃ/ phoneme in syllables into words. At the beginning of the semester, she was unable to correctly produce /ʃ/ in words. Currently, K. correctly produces /ʃ/ in 90% of her attempts.

The procedure used to meet objective 4 (monitoring of /ʃ/ in words) was K.'s use of ear training to locate her errors. She was required to stop immediately after each error in a word and self-correct it. Her monitoring ability in words has increased from 10% previously to 95% presently.

Objective 5 (production of /ʃ/ in phrases) was accomplished by having K. maintain her correct productions of /ʃ/ in words and integrate these words into phrases. Initially, K. was not able to correctly produce the /ʃ/ phoneme in phrases. Currently, she produces it correctly in 96% of her attempts.

Objective 6 (monitoring of /ʃ/ in phrases) was fulfilled by using ear training and self-correction. K. was asked to state whether or not each of her productions was correct. She was required to self-correct errors. Initially, K. was not able to monitor her productions in phrases. She now correctly monitors 90% of her productions.

Objective 7 (correct production of the /ʃ/ phoneme in conversation) was obtained by having K. engage in spontaneous conversation while concentrating on the proper production of the /ʃ/ phoneme. Her ability to correctly produce /ʃ/ in conversation has increased from 0% at the beginning of the semester to 96% currently.

To accomplish objective 8 (monitoring of the /ʃ/ phoneme in conversation), ear training and self-correction were used. K. was asked to correct any mistakes made on /ʃ/ in conversation immediately after they occurred. She was also told to anticipate any problems with producing /ʃ/ spontaneously and to prevent any distortions from

continues

Exhibit 4–8 continued

occurring. Her monitoring ability at the beginning of therapy was 10%. She is now able to monitor correctly 98% of her productions.

Results of Standardized Testing

The McDonald **Screening Deep Test of Articulation** was administered on February 4 and re-administered on May 7. The results of both tests were as follows:

	February	*May*
/s/ was correctly articulated in 10 of 10 contexts, or 100%		100%
/l/ was correctly articulated in 10 of 10 contexts, or 100%		100%
/r/ was correctly articulated in 10 of 10 contexts, or 100%		100%
/tʃ/ was correctly articulated in 1 of 10 contexts, or 10%		10%
/ʃ/ was correctly articulated in 0 of 10 contexts, or 0%		90%
/θ/ was correctly articulated in 10 of 10 contexts, or 100%		100%
/k/ was correctly articulated in 10 of 10 contexts, or 100%		100%
/f/ was correctly articulated in 10 of 10 contexts, or 100%		100%
/t/ was correctly articulated in 10 of 10 contexts, or 100%		100%

Correct productions of the /ʃ/ phoneme increased from 0% in February to 90% in May. Emphasis has not yet been placed on production of the /tʃ/ phoneme; therefore, the percentage of correct production remained the same.

The McDonald **Deep Test of Articulation** (sentence form) was also administered during February and May to reassess production of the /ʃ/ and /tʃ/ phonemes. K. correctly produced:

February

/tʃ/ as a releasor in 5 of 22 contexts, or in 23% of the attempts
/tʃ/ as an arrestor in 2 of 24 contexts, or in 8% of the attempts
/ʃ/   as a releasor in 0 of 22 contexts, or in 0% of the attempts
/ʃ/   as an arrestor in 0 of 24 contexts, or in 0% of the attempts

May

/tʃ/ as a releasor in 18 of 22 contexts, or in 82% of the attempts
/tʃ/ as an arrestor in 16 of 24 contexts, or in 67% of the attempts
/ʃ/   as a releasor in 20 of 22 contexts, or in 91% of the attempts
/ʃ/   as an arrestor in 23 of 24 contexts, or in 96% of the attempts

continues

Exhibit 4–8 continued

Improvement was noted from February to May on production of the /ʃ/ phoneme as both a releasor and arrestor. Improvement was also noted on production of /tʃ/ in both releasing and arresting positions.

Current Status and Impressions

Although progress was evident this semester, K.'s initial diagnosis of a mild articulation problem characterized by distortions of the /tʃ/ and /ʃ/ phonemes remain correct. Prognosis for further improvement is good based on her performance this semester, good attendance, active participation in therapy, and follow-through on all assignments.

Recommendations

K. P. should receive further remediation at the Maintown University's Speech and Hearing Center next fall. She should be seen individually twice a week for half-hour sessions. Therapeutic goals, pending re-evaluation due to summer vacation, may consist of the following:

1. to maintain correct production of /ʃ/ in conversation in 90% of her attempts
2. to maintain correct monitoring of /ʃ/ in conversation in 90% of her attempts
3. to correctly produce /tʃ/ in words in 90% of her attempts
4. to correctly monitor /tʃ/ in words in 90% of her attempts
5. to correctly produce /tʃ/ in words within phrases in 90% of her attempts
6. to correctly monitor productions of /tʃ/ in phrases in 90% of her attempts
7. to correctly produce /tʃ/ in conversation in 90% of her attempts
8. to correctly monitor productions of /tʃ/ in conversation in 90% of her attempts

Sally Storm
_____
Sally Storm
Undergraduate Student Clinician

Betty A. Brown, M.S. CCC/SLP
_____
Betty A. Brown, M.S. CCC/SLP
Clinical Supervisor

Exhibit 4–9 Sample Progress Report

[Identifying Information]

NAME: J. F.   FILE NUMBER:
ADDRESS: 00 Center Street   DATE: December 15 [this year]
                 Maintown, PA 19530   BIRTHDATE: January 19, [5 years ago]
PHONE: 000-000-0000   AGE: 5 years, 11 months
PARENTS: Jane and Bill   CLINICIAN: Jane Smith
PROBLEM: Language and   SEMESTER: Fall [this year]
                 Attending Behavior

PROGRESS REPORT

Background Information

   J. F., age 5 years, 11 months, received language therapy at the Maintown Medical Center from September 20 to December 15 this year. Services were provided by a student majoring in speech-language pathology at Maintown University. J. attended 19 of 22 sessions. He also receives physical and occupational therapy at Allville Speech Clinic in Allville, Pennsylvania, to remediate his developmental delays. J. received speech and language therapy last fall and spring semesters to remediate a moderate articulatory and language delay. For further information, please see the evaluation dated September 20.

Therapeutic Objectives

   J.'s therapeutic objectives for this semester were:

   1. to attend for 25 minutes in a structured therapy session
   2. to increase expressive vocabulary by 10 words
   3. to comprehend 5 prepositions of location and time in 90% of his attempts

Progress and Procedures

   Objective 1 (to attend for 25 minutes) was accomplished by using a variety of techniques. Sessions were held in a clutter-free environment and in as quiet an environment as possible. When extraneous noises distracted J. and he looked away, his

continues

Exhibit 4–9 continued

head was turned in the direction of the therapy materials and he was immediately reinforced verbally. The activities and materials used in a session were changed in order to maintain J.'s attention. Visual memory activities were used to increase J.'s attention and concentration. He was presented with two pictures that were then placed face down. The clinician pointed to a picture, and John named the picture that remained face down. This activity enabled J. to increase his visual memory such that he could name concealed pictures on three cards. J. is now able to attend for a 25-minute structured therapy session with only an occasional reminder to sit up and look at the therapeutic materials.

In order to accomplish objective 2 (increase expressive vocabulary by 10 words) the *World Book Dictionary* was consulted to obtain a list of age-appropriate words. The objective was accomplished using materials such as pictures, blocks, and puzzles. "Happy" and "sad" were explained using pictures and actual facial expressions. The client and clinician discussed items and occurrences that made J. happy. The shapes of blocks (square, round, triangle, rectangle) were explained using visual, auditory, and tactile senses. J. felt each shape in both hands to learn the concept of shapes. He first grouped and sorted blocks of similar shape, and he also receptively identified the shapes. Expressive identification of the shapes of the blocks is sporadic, but when J. is motivated he is able to name the different shapes appropriately. Words expressing qualities (hot, cold, empty, full) were emphasized during play situations. When J. washed his hands, the difference between hot and cold water was discussed. J. is able to receptively identify hot and cold water, but he expressively identifies all water as "hot." "Empty" and "full" were explained using boxes of blocks and puzzles that have individual pieces. J. learned that the spaces without a puzzle piece were "empty" and when the puzzle was completed, it was "full." He also removed all the blocks from a box to make it "empty" and replaced them to make it "full." The concept of "another" was explained while J. built with blocks and drew happy face cards. Whenever he wanted another card, he had to ask for it using the word "another." J. uses these words correctly and spontaneously in the therapy session.

Objective 3 (comprehension of locative and time prepositions) was accomplished using play therapy including blocks, trucks, and farm animals. "Before," "behind," "after," "in," and "under" were emphasized. J. was exposed to the locative prepositions in play activities where he was told to "put the block behind the cow" or "put the block in the dump truck" and "make the truck go behind the dump truck." "Under" was illustrated using a sheet and various toys, placing everything under the sheet. J. put blocks "in" the box, "under" chairs, and "behind" chairs. The concept of "before" was explained using sequencing puzzles such as building a snowman. J. also looked at pairs of pictures and pointed to the one that came before. J. comprehends these prepositions in 90% of his attempts.

continues

Exhibit 4–9 continued

Results of Testing

Receptive Language

The **Utah Test of Language Development** was administered in September and again in December to formally assess J.'s receptive language ability. J. achieved a language age equivalent of 2 years, 10 months in September and an age equivalent of 3 years, 3 months in December. In September, J. was able to identify pictures of objects and actions and was able to follow two-step directions such as "point to your ears and touch your nose." J. is now able to follow simple three-step directions. He receptively identified the colors red, blue, and yellow. J. also recognized body parts on the doll, the clinician, and himself. J. did not have success on these latter items during the September testing.

Expressive Language

The **Utah Test of Language Development** was administered in September and again in December to assess formally J.'s expressive language ability. J. achieved a language age equivalent of 2 years, 10 months in the initial testing and 3 years, 3 months in the final testing. During the final testing, J. did not name colors, but he was able to name pictures of common objects. J. repeated three digits and four words in a complex sentence. The length of the utterances J. uses to communicate his needs has increased from "Go play now" to "We're going to play." Although progress was evident, J. is functioning at a level 2 years, 8 months below his chronological age.

Informal assessment of J.'s language ability reveals an increase in original spontaneous language such as greetings and questions. J. immediately says "hi" to those people he recognizes and says "bye" when they leave. He also asks many Wh-questions about things in the environment that distract him (e.g., Where you going? What's he doing?). J. occasionally initiated conversation about himself (e.g., I have my pictures at home. My mom's coming). He has been observed interacting with his classmates during free play as well as structured activity.

Current Status and Impressions

J.'s language ability in September was 2 years, 11 months below his chronological age and is now only 2 years, 8 months below his chronological age. J.'s attention span has improved, so he is able to concentrate on structured therapeutic activities for the duration of the session. J. continues to exhibit a moderate receptive and expressive language delay. Progress is evident, although it is slow. Prognosis for further improvement is good owing to J.'s good attendance, his improved attending behaviors, and his family's motivation, cooperation, and follow-through.

continues

Exhibit 4–9 continued

Recommendations

J. F. should continue to receive language therapy on an individual basis twice a week for half hour sessions. Objectives for next semester should focus on the following:

1. increasing the length of utterances
2. increasing spontaneous language
3. increasing expressive vocabulary

Jane Smith
_____

Jane Smith
Undergraduate Student Clinician

Betty A. Brown, M.S. CCC/SLP
_____

Betty A. Brown, M.S. CCC/SLP
Clinical Supervisor

KNOW IT! USE IT!

After reading this chapter, you should be able to:

1. write an evaluation with fewer than five corrections as determined by your supervisor.
2. write a re-evaluation with fewer than five corrections as determined by your supervisor.
3. write a progress report with fewer than five corrections as determined by your supervisor.

REFERENCE

Paul-Brown, D. (1994). Clinical record keeping in audiology and speech-language pathology. *Asha, 36,* 40–42.

CHAPTER 5

Progress Notes

CHAPTER HIGHLIGHTS

- *background information on progress notes*
- *writing progress notes*
- *analyzing progress notes*
- *problems to avoid while writing progress notes*

This chapter provides information and examples to help you write progress notes, which are also called daily logs. These will become part of the client's permanent file. Following a discussion of the functions of progress notes, examples are presented and analyzed. Samples of problematic progress note entries and suggestions for improvement are then provided.

BACKGROUND

Accurate records are needed to record therapy and ensure the integrity and accountability of the clinicians. Paul-Brown (1994) states, "clear and comprehensive records are necessary to justify the need for treatment, to document the effectiveness of that treatment, and to have a legal record of events" (p. 40). Cornett and Chabon (1988) further note that "progress notes provide a complete and continuous record of all contacts (e.g., phone calls, letters, observations, therapy services, cancellations, clients' expressions of satisfaction or complaints about therapy, clinicians' suggestions or referrals) with or on behalf of the client" (p. 106). The American Speech-Language-Hearing Association (ASHA) requires that "accurate and complete records are maintained for each client and are protected with respect to confidentiality" (ASHA, 1992, p. 64).

Knepflar and May (1992, p. 23) advise that good progress notes will usually include the following:

1. brief notes concerning specific clinical management techniques and materials used.
2. interpretation of how the patient responded and statements regarding the patient's progress.
3. suggestions or assignments given to the patient and, when appropriate, recommendations for the next session.

Although not all authorities agree on the necessity to include all of Knepflar and May's suggestions in every progress note entry, each entry must at the minimum include the client's performance on each of the objectives. There is no standard length for a progress note entry. Although it has to be accurate and complete, it does not have to be long. The number of objectives worked on during a particular therapy session is a good predictor of the length of the entry. A progress note entry addressing a client's performance on two objectives should not be as long as one including performance on five objectives.

Progress notes must be objective rather than subjective. That is, they must be based on observable and verifiable behaviors rather than on personal reflections, feelings, prejudices, or perceptions. Paul-Brown (1994) states that with regard to clinical records, one should enter "only what has taken place, not anticipated activities or observations" (p. 42).

Each progress note entry should be dated for the day the therapy session was conducted, *not* the date the entry was written (it is recommended that entries should always be written on the day of the session). In addition, each entry should be signed except when more than one entry appears on a page. In this case, the first entry should be signed and all other entries on that page can be initialed. For organizational purposes, each page should be numbered. If you are making entries on both sides of the paper, it is less confusing if the front and back of each page has either a different number (1, 2, . . .) or a different letter following the same number (1A, 1B, . . .).

Each progress note entry should be self-contained. It should be understood without reading the progress note preceding or following it. The note should not refer the reader to other entries.

Writing progress notes is not an end in and of itself. Progress notes should be scrutinized to determine the flow and direction of the therapeutic program. It should be possible to understand the therapeutic regimen just by looking at and comparing the client's performance on each objective across sessions. Questions such as these should be answered: "Is the client having success?" "If so, is it appropriate to increase the complexity of the task?" "Is the client not performing successfully?" "If not, is it appropriate to continue to work on that objective?" "Should a different procedure be utilized?" "Is a branch step necessary?" "Is the objective not appropriate at this time?" If the client is performing successfully on an objective, the complexity should be increased.

Success is measured by whether or not the client has met the criterion, which is usually, but not always, set at correct performance in 90% of the attempts. Sometimes, this 90% criterion must be achieved in two or three consecutive sessions. Likewise, if the client is not performing successfully, the complexity should be decreased. If the client does not perform successfully on a particular objective, it is necessary to determine why. Perhaps the complexity is still too difficult, or perhaps the objective is not appropriate for the client at this time. In any case, it is necessary to make changes in the therapeutic program. At times, it is appropriate for progress notes to include the types of errors made when a client is not successful. It is often possible to gain insight by analyzing the client's errors or error patterns. Progress note entries can also be used to examine the response rate and determine whether it is adequate or needs to be increased.

Progress notes can follow different formats. Although the objectives and the client's performance must be provided, performance can be stated either in sentence form or by simply stating the results. This latter format does not use any more words than necessary. Sometimes a charting format is used. The actual format used is left to the discretion of the supervisor.

CUMULATIVE PROGRESS NOTE ENTRIES: SAMPLE

This client was 6 years, 1 month at the time the initial entry was made. A phonological problem of moderate severity was diagnosed. The processes of deletion of final consonants and cluster reduction constitute the focus. This client was expected to meet a criterion of 90% correct on two consecutive days before advancing in therapy. These entries do not reflect the beginning of the client's therapy program. Objective numbers do not remain constant and are numbered according to the order of focus within the session. These progress note entries are written in narrative form. Twelve consecutive sessions are critiqued. It is not necessary to number the sessions when writing progress notes; however, it was done here for the sole purpose of providing ease of reference for the analysis that appears later in this chapter. It does not seem necessary to state the nature of the errors made in this particular case, as they are either the use of open syllables or cluster reduction depending on which objective is emphasized. This information was clearly stated in the initial entries. (In the entries that follow, the objective appears first and is then followed by the client's performance.)

Session 1

- 3/20/[year]

- Objective 1:   Tom will close syllables on spontaneously produced monosyl-labic target words in 90% of his attempts.
- He closed syllables on 16 of 20 monosyllabic target words (80%). When a cloze procedure was used, he closed syllables in 14 of 20 attempts (70%).

- Objective 2:   Tom will correctly imitate the consonant clusters /st/, /sk/, and /sp/ when a pause is evident between the two consonants.
- He correctly imitated /s/+/t/ in 6 of 8 attempts (75%); /s/ and /k/ in 5 of 8 attempts (63%); and /s/+/p/ in 7 of 8 attempts (88%).

- 3/22/[year]–4/3/[year] Spring Break. Client did not receive services.

Session 2

- 4/4/[year]

- Objective 1:   Tom will close syllables on spontaneously produced monosyl-labic target words in 90% of his attempts.
- He closed syllables in 24 of 25 target words (96%). When a cloze procedure was used, he closed syllables in 18 of 20 attempts (90%).

- Objective 2:   Tom will correctly imitate the consonant clusters /st/, /sk/, and /sp/ when a pause is evident between the two consonants.
- He correctly imitated /s/+/t/ in 7 of 8 attempts (88%); /s/ and /k/ in 6 of 8 attempts (75%); and /s/+/p/ in 8 of 8 attempts (100%).

Session 3

- 4/7/[year]

- Objective 1:   Tom will close syllables on spontaneously produced monosyl-labic target words in 90% of his attempts.
- He closed syllables on all 25 target words (100%). When a cloze procedure was used, he closed syllables in 19 of 20 attempts (95%).

- <u>Objective 2</u>: Tom will close syllables on spontaneously produced monosyllabic target words in a carrier phrase in 90% of his attempts.
- He closed syllables on 35 of 45 monosyllabic target words in a carrier phrase (78%).

- <u>Objective 3</u>: Tom will correctly imitate the consonant clusters /st/, /sk/, and /sp/ when a pause is evident between the two consonants in 90% of his attempts.
- He correctly imitated /s/ and /t/ in 9 of 10 attempts (90%); /s/ and /k/ in 8 of 10 attempts (80%); and /s/ and /p/ in 9 of 10 attempts (90%).

Session 4

- 4/9/[year]

- <u>Objective 1</u>: Tom will close syllables on spontaneously produced monosyllabic target words in a carrier phrase in 90% of his attempts.
- He closed syllables in 50 of 55 attempts (91%).

- <u>Objective 2</u>: Tom will correctly imitate the consonant clusters /st/ and /sk/ when a pause is evident between the two consonants in 90% of his attempts.
- He correctly imitated /s/ and /t/ in 18 of 20 attempts (90%) and /s/ and /k/ in 23 of 24 attempts (96%).

- <u>Objective 3</u>: Tom will correctly imitate the consonant clusters /st/ and /sp/ in isolation without a pause in 90% of his attempts.
- He correctly imitated /st/ in 16 of 20 attempts (80%) and /sp/ in 17 of 20 attempts (85%).

Session 5

- 4/10/[year]

- <u>Objective 1</u>: Tom will close syllables on spontaneously produced monosyllabic target words in a carrier phrase in 90% of his attempts.
- He closed syllables in 40 of 42 attempts (95%).

- <u>Objective 2</u>: Tom will close syllables on monosyllabic target words in spontaneously produced phrases in 90% of his attempts.

- He closed syllables on 13 of 20 monosyllabic target words (65%) in spontaneously produced phrases.

- Objective 3:   Tom will correctly imitate the consonant cluster /sk/ when a pause is evident between the two consonants in 90% of his attempts.
- He correctly imitated /s/ and /k/ in 19 of 20 attempts (95%).

Session 6

- 4/11/[year]

- Objective 1:   Tom will close syllables on monosyllabic target words in spontaneously produced phrases in 90% of his attempts.
- He closed syllables on 27 of 36 monosyllabic target words (75%) in spontaneously produced phrases.

- Objective 2:   Tom will correctly imitate the consonant clusters /st/, /sk/, and /sp/ in isolation without a pause in 90% of his attempts.
- He correctly imitated /st/ in 9 of 10 attempts (90%); /sk/ in 14 of 15 attempts (93%); and /sp/ in 18 of 20 attempts (90%).

Session 7

- 4/14/[year]

- Objective 1:   Tom will close syllables on monosyllabic target words in spontaneously produced phrases in 90% of his attempts.
- Tom closed syllables on 20 of 25 monosyllabic target words in spontaneously produced phrases (80%).

- Objective 2:   Tom will correctly imitate the consonant clusters /st/, /sk/, and /sp/ without a pause in 90% of his attempts.
- He correctly imitated /st/ in 18 of 20 attempts (90%); /sk/ in 9 of 10 attempts (90%); and /sp/ in 24 of 25 attempts (96%).

- Objective 3:   Tom will correctly imitate the consonant clusters /st/, /sk/, and /sp/ in the initial position of words in 90% of his attempts.
- He correctly imitated /st/ in 7 of 10 words (70%); /sk/ in 6 of 10 words (60%); and /sp/ in 8 of 10 words (80%).

Session 8

- 4/17/[year]
- <u>Objective 1:</u>   Tom will close syllables on monosyllabic target words in spontaneously produced phrases in 90% of his attempts.
- Tom closed syllables on 18 of 22 monosyllabic target words in spontaneously produced phrases (82%).

- <u>Objective 2:</u>   Tom will correctly imitate the consonant clusters /st/, /sk/, and /sp/ in the initial position of words in 90% of his attempts.
- He correctly imitated /st/ in all 10 attempts (100%); /sk/ in 7 of 10 attempts (70%); and /sp/ in 9 of 10 attempts (90%).

Session 9

- 4/19/[year]
- <u>Objective 1:</u>   Tom will close syllables on monosyllabic target words in spontaneously produced phrases in 90% of his attempts.
- Tom closed syllables on 18 of 20 monosyllabic target words in spontaneously produced phrases (90%).

- <u>Objective 2:</u>   Tom will correctly imitate the consonant clusters /st/, /sk/, and /sp/ in the initial position of words in 90% of his attempts.
- He correctly imitated /st/ in all 12 attempts (100%); /sk/ in 16 of 20 attempts (80%); and /sp/ in 14 of 15 attempts (93%).

- <u>Objective 3:</u>   Tom will correctly spontaneously produce the consonant clusters /st/ and /sp/ in the initial position of words in 90% of his attempts.
- He correctly produced /st/ in the initial position of 6 of 10 words (60%) and /sp/ in 7 of 10 words (70%).

Session 10

- 4/22/[year]
- <u>Objective 1:</u>   Tom will close syllables on monosyllabic target words in spontaneously produced phrases in 90% of his attempts.
- Tom closed syllables on 25 of 26 monosyllabic target words in spontaneously produced phrases (96%).

- Objective 2:   Tom will close syllables on all words in spontaneously produced phrases in 90% of his attempts.
- He closed syllables on 8 of 10 words (80%) in spontaneously produced
  phrases.

- Objective 3:   Tom will correctly imitate the consonant cluster /sk/ in the initial position of words in 90% of his attempts.
- He correctly imitated /sk/ in the initial position of 18 of 20 attempts (90%).

- Objective 4:   Tom will correctly spontaneously produce the consonant cluster /st/ and /sp/ in the initial position of words in 90% of his
  attempts.
- He correctly produced /st/ in the initial position of 9 of 10 words (90%) and
  /sp/ in 18 of 20 words (90%).

Session 11

- 4/25/[year]

- Objective 1:   Tom will close syllables on all words in spontaneously produced phrases in 90% of his attempts.
- He closed syllables on 18 of 20 words in spontaneously produced phrases
  (90%).
- Objective 2:   Tom will correctly imitate the consonant cluster /sk/ in the initial position of words in 90% of his attempts.
- He correctly imitated the consonant cluster /sk/ in the initial position of all 10
  words (100%).
- Objective 3:   Tom will correctly spontaneously produce the consonant clusters /st/, /sk/, and /sp/ in the initial position of words in 90% of
  his attempts.
- He correctly produced /st/ in 19 of 20 words (95%); /sk/ in 6 of 10 words
  (60%); and /sp/ in 9 of 10 words (90%).

Session 12

- 4/27/[year]

- Objective 1:   Tom will close syllables on all words in spontaneously produced phrases in 90% of his attempts.

- Tom closed syllables on 45 of 48 words (94%) in spontaneously produced phrases.

- Objective 2:   Tom will correctly spontaneously produce the consonant cluster /sk/ in the initial position of words in 90% of his attempts.
- He correctly produced /sk/ in 28 of 40 words (70%).

- Objective 3:   Tom will correctly spontaneously produce the consonant clusters /st/ and /sp/ in the initial position of words in sentences in 90% of his attempts.
- He correctly produced /st/ in the initial position of 8 of 10 words in sentences (80%) and /sp/ in 12 of 16 words in sentences (75%).

- 4/29/[year] Canceled due to client illness

CUMULATIVE PROGRESS NOTE ENTRIES: ANALYSIS

Objective: Addition of Final Consonants

The progress note entries shown in the previous section will now be analyzed and discussed to determine whether the flow and direction of the therapeutic program is sound. It is important to note again that the criterion is correct usage in 90% of the attempts and that this criterion must be achieved on two consecutive days. Our first focus will be on the objective, "Tom will close syllables on spontaneously produced monosyllabic target words. . . ." This objective was worked on in session 1, but the criterion was not met. The criterion was met in session 2. Because the criterion had to be met on two consecutive days, this objective remained a focus during session 3. The criterion was again met. Therefore a new, related but more complex, objective was introduced. It is, "Tom will close syllables on spontaneously produced monosyllabic target words in a carrier phrase . . . ," which was introduced during the latter portion of session 3. The criterion was not met in this session, but it was met in sessions 4 and 5. The complexity of this task was then increased by changing the focus from carrier phrases to spontaneously produced phrases as seen in the objective, "Tom will close syllables on monosyllabic target words in spontaneously produced phrases . . . ," which was introduced in session 5. The criterion was not met in sessions 5, 6, 7, or 8. However, improvement in performance can be seen (65%, 75%, 80%, and 82%, respectively). The criterion was met in sessions 9 and 10. Therefore, the task was again increased in complexity, as seen in the next objective, and was introduced during the latter portion of session

10: "Tom will close syllables on all words in spontaneously produced phrases. . . ." The criterion was not met during session 10, but it was met during the next two sessions (sessions 11 and 12). A further increase in complexity is now warranted. Although additional sessions were not provided in the progress note entries, realistic future objectives could consist of the following: "Tom will close syllables on all words in spontaneously produced sentences," "Tom will close syllables on all words spoken during 30 seconds of conversation," and "Tom will close syllables on all words spoken during 1 minute of conversation," respectively. If believed necessary, reading could be incorporated between the focus on sentences and conversation.

Objective: Cluster Production

Our focus will be placed on the objective, "Tom will correctly imitate the consonant clusters /st/, /sp/, and /sk/ when a pause is evident between the two consonants . . . ," which was introduced in session 1. The criterion was not met on any of the clusters during this session (75%, 63%, and 88%, respectively). Criterion was met for the first time on /sp/ (100%) in session 2, but not on /st/ (88%) or /sk/ (75%). Criterion was met for the second time on /sp/ and for the first time on /st/ (90%) in session 3. The criterion was met for the second time on /st/ in session 4. Therefore, it was appropriate to again increase the complexity on /sp/ and /st/ during the latter part of session 4. However, /sk/ was worked on first, and the criterion was met (96%) for the first time. Therefore the next objective, "Tom will correctly imitate the consonant clusters /st/ and /sp/ in isolation without a pause . . . ," was introduced. The criterion was not met on either cluster during this session. The cluster /sk/ was still being worked on with a pause between the consonants, and the criterion was met for the second time (95%) in session 5. Therefore, all three clusters imitated without a pause could be emphasized in session 6. The criterion was met for the first time on all three clusters during this session and for the second time during session 7. Therefore, the complexity was again increased, as can be seen in the objective, "Tom will correctly imitate the consonant clusters /st/, /sp/, and /sk/ in the initial position of words. . . ." The criterion was not met on any of the clusters during this session, but was met on /st/ (100%) and /sp/ (90%) for the first time during session 8 and for the second time during session 9 (100% and 93%, respectively). During the latter half of session 9, the objective, "Tom will correctly spontaneously produce the consonant clusters /st/ and /sp/ in the initial position of words . . ." was introduced. The criterion was not met in this session, but it was met in both sessions 10 and 11. Because the objective, "to imitate the consonant cluster /sk/ in the initial position of words . . ." met the criterion in sessions 10 and 11, /sk/ was also included with /st/ and /sp/ in the objective, "spontaneous production in the initial position of words . . ." during the latter part of session 11. The clusters /st/ and /sp/ had already met the criterion in session 10 and did so again in session 11. The criterion was not met on /sk/ during session 11. Because criterion was met on /st/ and /sp/, complexity on these two clusters was again increased. The new objective, "Tom will correctly spontaneously produce the consonant clusters /st/ and /sp/ in the initial position of words in sentences . . ." was introduced in session 12. Criterion was not met during this session.

Conclusion

In analyzing Tom's performance, it is apparent that the objectives were appropriate. They were not so easy that he was immediately successful. They were not so difficult that success could not be attained. The objectives were appropriately graded in complexity in that each was slightly more difficult than the preceding one. Success on a preceding objective was necessary for all following objectives. Analysis of the progress note entries enables one to conclude that the flow and direction of the therapeutic program was appropriate for this client. All of these points are reflected in these progress notes as they should be. Progress notes that are not well written are neither clear nor useful, as you shall see.

QUICK CHECK

After writing a progress note entry, make certain it follows from the previous entry. Compare entries to make certain progress is evident on a particular objective. Use the information recorded in your progress notes to help guide you in further planning the client's therapy program.

PROBLEMATIC ENTRIES

Several examples of progress note entries that are problematic in some aspect(s) are now presented and discussed. Problematic entries are set in boldface. Revisions are simply highlighted. Entries are not based on the same client, therefore there is no continuity between or among entries.

Problem 1: No Objective Stated

11/13/[year]   Mary did not meet the objective.

- **/b/ 17/20 = 85%**
- **/d/ 17/20 = 85%**
- **/g/ 15/20 = 75%**

Mary was tired today. However, she watched me carefully as I produced the sounds in CV (consonant–vowel) combinations in the mirror.

Discussion and Revision

The objective was never stated. On the basis of the commentary, the objective can be hypothesized, but this runs the risk of being misconstrued. Many readers would get the impression that the client is spontaneously producing the phonemes, when in fact the client is imitating. The statement, "Mary was tired today," is subjective. An acceptable revision is:

11/13/[year]   The objective is to imitate the /b/, /d/, and /g/ phonemes correctly in CV combinations. Results:

- */b/ 17/20 = 85%*
- */d/ 17/20 = 85%*
- */g/ 15/20 = 75%*

Mary yawned 10 times and put her head on the table twice during this session.

QUICK CHECK

Always make certain that the objective is clearly stated in each progress note entry.

Problem 2: No Objective and Client's Performance Ignored

11/20/[year]   Four objectives were attempted. The results are review of imitation on two-syllable words 5/10 (50%); production of two-syllable words 4/10 (40%); imitation of three-syllable words 2/10 (20%); and production of three-syllable words 1/10 (10%). Criterion was not met on any objective.

Discussion and Revision

The objective again is not stated, but it can be inferred. The biggest problem inherent in this entry involves ignoring the client's performance. The client did not meet the criterion on the review, which was imitation of two-syllable words, which was the least complex objective attempted during this session. Because the client did not have success imitating two-syllable words, there should not have been any progression to the production of two-syllable words, let alone imitation and production of three-syllable words, which are all not only more complex but naturally build on the less complex objective. This clearly is an example of not letting the client's performance guide clinical decisions. In this case, decreasing the complexity of the task, not increasing it, would have been appropriate. An acceptable revision is:

11/20/[year]   *The first objective is to correctly imitate two-syllable words. David did so on 5 of 10 words (50%). This task was then modified. As each word was presented, the clinician tapped each syllable on the table. David correctly imitated both the word and the tapping in 9 of 10 attempts (90%). The next task consisted of the clinician saying the words, but not tapping. David correctly imitated the production and tapped the syllables on his own in 8 of 10 attempts (80%) on his first trial and 10 of 10 attempts (100%) on his second trial. David then imitated 18 of 20 two syllable words (90%) without tapping.*

QUICK CHECK

Make certain the client's performance is your guide. This record should help you determine whether the therapeutic focus is appropriate or if it needs to be changed or modified.

Problem 3: Data Incomplete

2/15/[year]   **John will correctly produce /n, p, f, k, d, b, g/ in the initial position of words in 90% of his attempts.**

Result: 36/40

Discussion and Revision

On the surface, the entry just shown looks well written. The objective is clearly stated as is the result. The percentage was omitted, but 36 of 40 is 90%, so the criterion was met. It is, however, best to keep separate data and record results on each phoneme so that problematic areas are not masked. In actuality, the results were /n/ 5 of 5 (100%); /p/ 5 of 5 (100%); /f/ 6 of 6 (100%); /k/ 6 of 6 (100%); /d/ 4 of 8 (50%); /b/ 5 of 5 (100%); and /g/ 5 of 5 (100%). Note that John did not have success on the phoneme /d/. When cumulative results were provided (36 of 40), however, it appeared that the criterion was met. It was, but only on 6 of the 7 phonemes. In other words, the specific results on each phoneme were masked. It would be unfair to the client to expect him to function on a higher level on the /d/ phoneme, which would be the next step in his therapeutic program. An acceptable revision is:

2/15/[year]   John will correctly produce /n, p, f, k, d, b, g/ in the initial position of words in 90% of his attempts.

Results:
- /n/ 5 of 5 (100%)
- /p/ 5 of 5 (100%)
- /f/ 6 of 6 (100%)
- /k/ 6 of 6 (100%)
- /d/ 4 of 8 (50%)
- /b/ 5 of 5 (100%)
- /g/ 5 of 5 (100%)

QUICK CHECK

Be as accountable as possible! Provide data for each objective as well as for each part of each objective in your progress note entries.

Problem 4: Ambiguity

10/25/[year] Sally will auditorially and tactually discriminate between voiced and voiceless phonemes during 90% of her attempts.

Results:
- 35 trials
- 63%

Sally was bored at times. She had difficulty sitting properly on her chair. Her attention span was extremely short.

Discussion and Revision

Either the voiced and voiceless cognate pairs should have been listed, or the objective should have read "between all voiced and voiceless phonemes." Otherwise, the phonemes included are ambiguous. The client attempted 35 trials, but the number correct was not stated. Because the client was only successful on 63% of her attempts, the errors should have been listed. More information is necessary. The clinician should have included the client's performance on each phoneme, as this is most beneficial for designing the therapeutic program. The last three statements in the entry are subjective. An acceptable revision is:

10/25/[year] Sally will auditorially and tactually discriminate between the voiced and voiceless phonemes /p, b, t, d, k, g, f, v/ during 90% of her attempts.

Results:
- */p/ 8 of 10 (80%)*
- */b/ 6 of 10 (60%)*
- */t/ 9 of 10 (90%)*
- */d/ 7 of 10 (70%)*
- */k/ 8 of 10 (80%)*
- */g/ 6 of 10 (60%)*
- */f/ 7 of 10 (70%)*
- */v/ 6 of 10 (60%)*

Overall results:
- *voiced 32 of 40 (80%)*
- *voiceless 25 of 40 (63%)*

Errors: Sally stated that 8 voiced phonemes were voiceless and 15 voiceless phonemes were voiced.
Sally frequently looked out the window— eight times during the session. She got up

out of her chair four times during this session. The longest she attended to a task today was 3 minutes.

QUICK CHECK

Upon completion of your progress note entries, reread them. Make certain to provide as much information as possible about the client's performance. Everyone reading your entries should be able to interpret them in the manner in which you intended.

Problem 5: Wrong Emphasis

2/16/[year] **Today's session consisted of elicitation of the /s/ and /z/ phonemes in monologue. The client was required to describe visual stimuli provided by the clinician in the form of <u>Verb Action Picture Cards</u> while correctly producing the target phonemes in continuous speech. James correctly produced the target phonemes with the following results:**

- **/s/ 34 of 36 attempts (94%)**
- **/z/ 33 of 36 attempts (92%)**

The clinician provided a verbal prompt upon presentation of each stimulus picture, such as "Tell me what the girl is doing" or "What is the boy wearing?". James is constantly able to monitor his speech during monologue as evidenced by his frequency of self-corrections without the presence of a model. The client must continue to be reminded to monitor his speech during informal conversation with the clinician.

Discussion and Revision

One problem intrinsic to this entry is that the focus appears to be on the clinician more so than on the client. In the opening sentence, "Today's session consisted of elicitation of the /s/ and /z/ phonemes in monologue," it is the clinician who elicits and the client who produces. Therefore, the emphasis should be placed on the client. Meeting the criterion should not directly depend on the clinician's elicitation but on the client's production. There are three additional unnecessary references to the clinician. Further, stating the specific stimulus materials used, *Verb Action Picture Cards,* is not necessary because it does not serve any purpose in this particular entry. It is not a particular program being followed. With further analysis, the objective that appears to be production of stated phonemes in monologue was not even attempted. Answering questions such as "Tell me what the girl is doing?" or "What is the boy wearing?" does not engage the client in monologue, but instead, the client produces responses to specific questions within a structured situation. Stating "while correctly producing the target phonemes in continuous speech" is misleading for the reasons already given. Lack of accountability is evident regarding James's ability to "monitor his speech during monologue as evidenced by his frequency of self-corrections without the presence of a model." How accurate is his monitoring? How many self-corrections were made? To be accountable, these questions must be addressed and answered.

It is difficult to revise the entry shown because the objective is not clearly stated, and, upon analysis, as already stated, it is ambiguous. Is the objective "James will correctly produce the /s/ and /z/ phonemes while answering specific questions in 90% of his attempts" or is it "James will correctly produce the /s/ and /z/ phonemes during monologue in 90% of his attempts"? Because of the ambiguity, the entry will be revised reflecting both of these possible objectives. An acceptable revision for the first interpretation is:

> 2/16/[year]   *The objective was correct production of /s/ and /z/ while answering specific questions ("What is the girl doing?" "What is the boy wearing?").*
>
> *Results:*
> - */s/ 34 of 36 (94%)*
> - */z/ 33 of 36 (92%)*
>
> *James monitored all 72 productions correctly (100%) and self-corrected 4 of his 5 erred productions (80%).*

An acceptable revision for the second interpretation is:

> 2/16/[year]   *The objective (James will correctly produce the /s/ and /z/ phonemes in monologue) was accomplished*

by having James select three topics to discuss. While talking, he correctly produced the /s/ phoneme in 34 of 36 attempts (94%) and /z/ in 33 of 36 attempts (92%). He correctly monitored all 72 productions (100%) and self-corrected 4 of his 5 errors (80%).

QUICK CHECK

Remember that the client is the recipient of your therapy. State all objectives in your progress note entries in terms of what the client will do, not what you will do.

SUBJECTIVE, OBJECTIVE, ASSESSMENT, AND PLAN FORMAT

A familiar format for problem oriented progress notes is the SOAP format (Hegde and Davis, 1995). SOAP is an acronym for subjective, objective, assessment, and plan. The frequency with which SOAP notes are written varies. Some settings require one SOAP note to be written for the week regardless of the number of therapy sessions rendered. Other settings require one SOAP note to be written per therapy session. Each part of SOAP is addressed separately here.

Subjective

This part includes subjective observations. Impressions of the client's behavior are described in this part of the progress note. These impressions can be the client's, the clinician's, or the family's. Use direct quotes to support statements when possible. Examples are:

Mary appeared upset today. She stated, "My best friend isn't talking to me."

―――――

Jimmy's mother is pleased. She said, "Jimmy is talking so much better!"

―――――

Sally looked better today. Her nurse stated, "She's very alert today."

Use facts to support statements if possible. For example: "Johnny is very motivated. Instead of finding 10 objects that begin with /s/, he found 20."

Objective

Measurable information is included in the objective section. State your goal in a behavioral objective format and then indicate the client's performance. If applicable, compare the client's performance with that of his previous session. For example:

> *Johnny will correctly produce /s/ in the initial position of words in 90% of his attempts. He correctly produced /s/ in the initial position of words in 30 of 40 attempts (75%) as compared with 25 of 40 (63%) last session. A 12% improvement is evident.*

Another example is:

> *Jimmy will spontaneously use noun + verb combinations eight times during the session. Today, he spontaneously produced six noun + verb combinations compared with three during the last session.*

Test results are also included in this section of the progress note (Flower, 1984).

Assessment

In this section, assess your objective data. This is where you briefly summarize the data. If possible, make a statement regarding the severity of the problem. For example:

> *The client presents with a severe phonological process problem. It is characterized by consistent usage of deletion of final consonants, fronting, and stopping.*

This section also includes the client performance. Strengths as well as weaknesses may be discussed. Hypotheses for why change did or did not occur may also be included.

Plan

The course of treatment is outlined in the plan section. Specifically state the therapy goals for the next session (or week) depending on the frequency with which progress notes are written. These goals also include future diagnostic goals if applicable. All goals must be written in a behavioral objective format. New goals should stem from the client's performance on the previous therapy goals. Examples are:

> *Johnny will correctly produce /s/ in the initial position of words in 90% of his attempts.*

> *Johnny will correctly imitate /s/ in the final position of words in 70% of his attempts.*

Another example is:

> *Jimmy will spontaneously use noun + verb combinations in 90% of the obligatory contexts.*

Ways of Writing

The SOAP format can be written in various ways. Two ways will be demonstrated. One way shows a clear delineation between the *S, O, A,* and *P* portions. An example is:

> *7/19/[year]*
> - *S: Joe appeared happy today. He smiled frequently throughout the session.*
> - *O: He correctly imitated 20 of 25 (80%) monosyllabic words beginning with /s/. He correctly produced 45 of 50 (90%) words beginning with /l/ in phrases. Joe demonstrated progress on both phonemes today. The production of /s/ increased from 65% to 80% and /l/ from 75% to 90%.*
> - *A: Joe continues to present with an articulation problem of moderate severity.*
> - *P: Continue current treatment goals and activities next session.*

The second way uses a narrative format. Although the parts are not clearly visible, the information is presented in the established order of subjective, objective, assessment, and plan. An example is:

> *7/19/[year]   Joe appeared happy today. He smiled frequently throughout the session. He correctly imitated 20 of 25 (80%) monosyllabic words beginning with /s/. He cor-*

rectly produced 45 of 50 (90%) words beginning with /l/ in phrases. Joe demonstrated progress on both phonemes today. Production of /s/ increased from 65% to 80% and /l/ from 75% to 90%. Joe continues to present with an articulation problem of moderate severity. Continue with current treatment goals and activities next session.

It is important to note that the same information is included in both entries. It is solely the format that varies.

QUICK CHECK

If you are using SOAP format, make certain that *subjective, objective, assessment,* and *plan* are all reflected in each progress note entry.

CONCLUSION

It is hoped that the information presented in this chapter will advance your understanding of the importance and usefulness of well-written progress notes. It is also hoped that the knowledge gained will enable you to write acceptable progress notes from the start. Further, the value of well-written progress notes can best be learned and truly understood in a situation when a client, previously seen by a fellow beginning clinician, is switched to your caseload mid-semester and progress notes are either lacking or sketchy at best. Nothing will reinforce the importance of well-written progress notes more quickly than finding yourself in this situation. It is hoped, however, that neither you nor your peers will be guilty of writing unacceptable progress note entries.

KNOW IT! USE IT!

After reading this chapter, you should be able to:

1. state how you can use your progress notes to help determine the flow and direction of the client's therapeutic program to the satisfaction of your supervisor
2. correctly write progress notes in 90% of your attempts as determined by your supervisor
3. state and explain in detail at least four problems that can occur when writing progress notes
4. correctly determine whether your progress notes are well written or problematic in 90% of your attempts
5. explain SOAP format in detail to your supervisor

REFERENCES

American Speech-Language-Hearing Association. (1992). Standards for professional service programs in speech-language pathology and audiology. *Asha, 34,* 63–70.

Cornett, B., & Chabon, S. (1988). *The clinical practice of speech-language pathology.* Columbus, OH: Merrill.

Flower, R. (1984). *Delivery of speech-language pathology and audiology services.* Baltimore, MD: Williams & Wilkins.

Hegde, M.N., & Davis, D. (1995). *Clinical methods and practicum in speech-language pathology* (2nd ed.). San Diego, CA: Singular.

Knepflar, K., & May, A. (1992). *Report writing in the field of communication disorders: A handbook for students and clinicians* (2nd ed.). Rockville, MD: National Student Speech Language Hearing Association.

Paul-Brown, D. (1994). Clinical record keeping in audiology and speech-language pathology. *Asha, 36,* 40–42.

CHAPTER 6

Taming the Paper Giant: Ensuring Accuracy and Accountability

CHAPTER HIGHLIGHTS

- *the importance of accountability*
- *an efficient system for handling paperwork*
- *record-keeping systems*
- *record-keeping during individual therapy sessions*
- *record-keeping during group therapy sessions*
- *tracking clinical hours*
- *ASHA's certification requirements*

One of the most valuable pieces of advice that can be given to you when you start clinical practicum is to stay on top of the paperwork from the very beginning. Many of you have heard this advice, but will all of you follow it? If you fall behind, you will soon find it is difficult to catch up. If you get caught in this situation, you will find yourself playing "catch-up" for the rest of the semester. For the most part, those of you who will follow this advice will likely have more positive clinical experiences. For those of you who ignore this tip, the end result will likely be negative clinical experiences, undesirable grades, or, in some cases, the need to retake the clinical experience (Figure 6–1).

To avoid this stumbling block, some of you may voice a desire to use one of the many computer programs that are available to assist with the administration of clinical functions. You may be tempted to use one or more programs in the belief that you will automatically become a better clinician. This is not necessarily true. It is my hope that this chapter will give you a better understanding of the "how" and "why" of the paperwork process. Later, when you understand the conceptual elements, you will be able to make an informed decision about the use of software.

This chapter also raises the sometimes sensitive topic of accountability and its link to the paperwork process. Leahy (1995) interprets accountability "as having

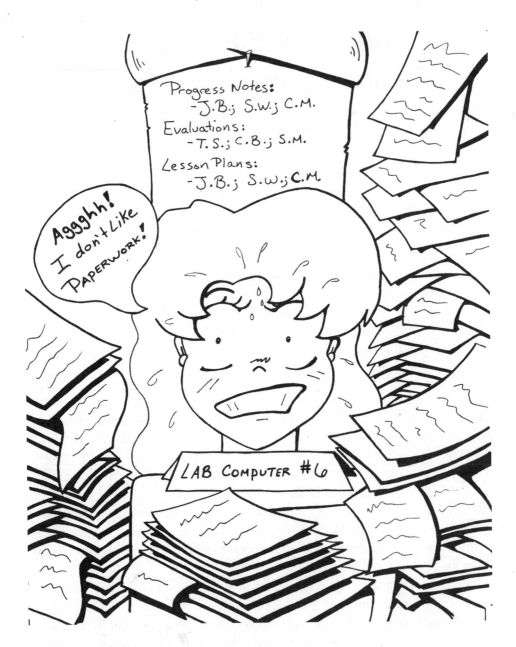

Figure 6–1 Death by paperwork.

readily accessible complete records of clients served, along with a justifiable ratio-nale to document need for service" (p. 88). Records are evidence of what will hap-pen or what has happened from initial contact through discharge from therapy.

Accurate records are essential to guide and shape the therapeutic regimen and to document client performance. The more accurate these records are, the fewer misinterpretations can occur over what was the intent and outcome of the clinician's work.

PAPERWORK PROCESS AND A SYSTEM FOR STREAMLINING

"Paperwork" is a relative term because the type of documents included frequently varies among service providers. There is, however, some consistency within collegiate programs. The writing of behavioral objectives, evaluations, reevaluations, lesson plans, session evaluations, progress notes, and progress reports (all are addressed in this book) are required by most programs. Although there are other documents used in speech-language pathology, this section focuses on those that are linked directly to the therapy session progress notes, lesson plans, session evaluations, and response sheets. An efficient and effective, or "streamlined," system is designed for handling these paperwork elements.

When a client is evaluated and therapy is recommended, a *semester plan of treatment* must be constructed. This plan is composed of both long-range goals and short-term objectives. The ideas and content for constructing this plan are based on formal and informal testing and observations made during the initial evaluation. The construction of this plan is the second step toward the implementation of therapy (the evaluation is the first step). A *lesson plan* is constructed before therapy begins. A lesson plan may be required for each session or one may cover all sessions held during an entire week. Although the frequency with which lesson plans are required varies, they all contain objectives for the session (short-term objectives) as well as the procedures (specific techniques, tasks, materials, and method of reinforcement) used to meet these objectives. In addition, many supervisors request a written rationale for each procedure.

The paperwork process does not end with the completion of a session. *Progress notes* need to be written. It is best to write them immediately following the session. The reason is that your mind and thoughts are still on the session and records containing data on the client's performance on the various therapeutic objectives are right at your fingertips. These data form the basis for your progress notes.

The clinician is now required to provide a detailed and insightful *evaluation* of the therapy session. This evaluation is usually written on the back of the lesson plan. It should likewise be written immediately following the session. Some aspects to be included in this analysis center on the objectives: "Were they met or not?" "What were the results?" Likewise, procedures are to be scrutinized: "Which procedures were helpful and which were not?" "Why?" "Was progress made?"

"Why or why not?" "If something did not go well, what could have been done differently?" "What were the strengths of the session?" "Why?" "What were the weaknesses?" "Why?" "What will be done differently during the next session?"

Now it seems that the paperwork is finished; however, it all starts over again for the next session. This is the point at which it is possible to streamline paperwork that is done for every session. In the same time frame, the following should be completed: progress notes and session evaluation for the session just completed, and a lesson plan and response sheet for the next session. Often, beginning clinicians look at these as being separate entities and move from one part of the paperwork process to another, whenever time is available. This is not the best approach because these records constitute a reporting "system" as shown in Table 6–1.

A streamlined way to tackle the paperwork is to do it immediately after conducting the therapy session. This is easier if you are organized and were actively thinking about and evaluating performance (both yours and the client's) during the session. Once this system is put into place, paperwork will be completed thoroughly and quickly. Under these conditions, the session evaluation, the progress notes, the lesson plan for the *next* session as well as the response sheet (discussed later in this chapter) for the *next* session can be completed in approximately 20 minutes.

If the progress notes and session evaluation for the current session, and lesson plan and response sheet for the next session, are done at four different times, efficiency decreases and time is wasted. This is because it will be necessary to rethink and review the previous therapy session four separate times—once before writing the session evaluation, once before writing the progress notes, once before writing the lesson plan for the next session, and yet again before designing the response sheet for the next session. This is not efficient because you will need to re-create the therapy set, and this takes more time than the actual writing. Keep in mind that the writing cannot be done unless your mind and thoughts are focused on the therapy session. If these four parts are completed immediately following the session, your mind and thoughts are *already* on that session.

QUICK CHECK

Make certain you are streamlining the paperwork process. Focus on one client at a time. Write your progress note immediately following the session. Then continue with your written evaluation of that same session. Next, get your lesson plan and response sheet written for your next session with this same client. By completing all the necessary paperwork for one client in the same time frame, efficiency is increased and time is used wisely.

Table 6–1 Steps in the Therapeutic Process and Paperwork Requirements

Therapy Stage and Recording Requirement	Frequency of Preparation	Documentary Requirement(s) (Partial List)
Pre-therapy Procedures		
Evaluation	Initially (and as ordered)	Testing (formal and informal) Observations
Plan of treatment	1 per semester (may be modified)	Long-range goals Short-term objectives
Lesson plan	1 per session (or week)	Short-term objectives Procedures Rationale (optional)
Response sheet(s)	1 (or more) per session	Performance on objectives
Therapy Session		
Post-therapy Procedures		
Progress notes	1 per session	Client's summarized performance
Session evaluation (becomes part of lesson plan)	1 per session	Were objectives met? Were procedures appropriate? Was session productive?
Lesson plan	1 for next session or week	Short-term objectives Procedures Rationale (optional)
Response sheet(s)	1 (or more) for next session	Performance on objectives

RECORD-KEEPING DURING INDIVIDUAL SESSIONS

It is known that excellent record-keeping does not guarantee good care, but poor record-keeping is an obstacle to clinical excellence (Kibbee & Lilly, 1989). It is necessary to keep accurate records. This can be done in a couple of ways when seeing clients for individual therapy sessions.

One such method consists of keeping continuous records during the entire therapy session. All relevant responses, those directed at the objectives, are recorded as long as the session is in progress. These data, in your records, then comprise the substance for progress notes. If records are not kept, it is not possible to write accurate objective progress notes.

When the recording of every response interferes with the naturalistic setting or impacts negatively on the flow of the session, another method of record-keeping must be implemented. This second method involves samplings of behaviors during the therapy session rather than the continuous recording of responses. Each objective should be targeted for record-keeping for a set time limit that you will determine. For example, if there are three objectives, you may decide to keep records on objective 1 for 2 minutes, objective 2 for 2 minutes, and so forth. Pending the nature of the objective, the 2-minute time frame should be limited to responses by the client.

One problem found with any record-keeping method is that beginning clinicians frequently neglect to record some responses, which results in inaccurate data. A few reasons for failing to record responses are getting too involved in the task at hand and simply forgetting, not realizing that a target response was attempted, not realizing that a target response was produced, or concentrating too much on what to do next rather than on what is being done at that moment. To increase the likelihood of recording all responses (continuous record-keeping) or all responses during the set time (sampling), a response sheet (record sheet, tally sheet, data sheet) should be set up prior to the session. This response sheet should be positioned so that responses or their outcomes can easily be recorded and you should place your pen or pencil point on the paper at the place where the next response should be written. If this sheet is within easy reach and if one's writing instrument remains in position, it will serve as a constant reminder to record the client's responses. This sheet should have each objective stated in abbreviated form with enough space available to keep a tally of responses. An example can be found in Exhibit 6–1.

Note that because objectives 1 and 2 were clearly defined at a previous time, the actual stimulus items are known before beginning the session. Therefore, it is possible to include the actual stimulus items on your response or tally sheet prior to the

Exhibit 6–1 Sample Response Sheet

Objective 1	*Objective 2*	*Objective 3*
(Receptive Identification)	*(Expressive Identification)*	*(Production of Is + Verbing)*
1. eye	1. eye	
2. ear	2. ear	
3. knee	3. knee	
4. hand	4. hand	
5. foot	5. foot	
6. mouth	6. mouth	
7. elbow	7. elbow	
8. chin	8. chin	
9. face	9. face	
10. finger	10. finger	

session. This saves time by eliminating the need to write them while the client's responses are occurring. The stimulus items in objective 3 cannot be formulated before the session because the client will be selecting a book and discussing actions of various people or animals. In such cases, the specific stimulus items cannot be predetermined. In this instance, it is best to write down simply that portion of the client's response that resembles the target structure (is + Verbing) as it is being produced. In this manner, it will be possible to analyze the client's responses further.

QUICK CHECK

Make certain you are keeping records on the client's responses. Decide whether you will use continuous record-keeping or sampling prior to the start of the session. Stick with it!

RECORD-KEEPING DURING GROUP SESSIONS

Compared with individual therapy, it is not always realistic or feasible to record all responses produced by each client on every objective during a group therapy session. This is especially true if three or more clients are in attendance and/or the session is actually one of *group therapy* as opposed to *therapy in groups* (as discussed in chapter 7). Nevertheless, it is still necessary to keep records because accountability is required. This is a situation, however, in which continuous record-keeping of all responses for all clients is simply not possible. The sampling method previously discussed is a feasible alternative.

To keep records in a group setting, record each client's responses for only one or two objectives targeted for that particular session. If the size of the group is large (five or six clients), it will not be possible to record responses for each child during each session. If this is the case, target objectives for half the clients for one session and then target the rest of the clients the next session.

If a client is working on more than two objectives, those targeted should change for each session in order to compensate for the limits imposed by the group setting. Ideally, each objective should be targeted at least every week and a half. This frequency will vary pending the number of sessions each client receives per week, the number of clients present during a session, and the length of the session. This sampling approach is acceptable when recording all responses produced by each client during each session is not possible (Figure 6–2).

QUICK CHECK

Make certain you have adequate records for all children in the group and all objectives worked on over a realistic length of time.

RECORD-KEEPING WITH YOUNG OR VERY ACTIVE CHILDREN

Many students have stated that it is difficult to keep records during sessions in which they are manipulating lots of materials in an attempt to keep the children's interest or in sessions in which they are following the child's lead. This frequently requires the clinician to move around the room with the child and frequently to be on the floor with the child. This does present a difficulty with keeping records in the conventional manner—making marks on a sheet of paper either located on the table or that you are carrying as you move around during the session. There is a better way. Self-adhesive paper can be stuck on the nondominant arm, and records can be kept in this fashion. Tape can also be used in this same manner. As long as you have a pen or pencil handy, record-keeping in these situations should no longer be problematic.

QUICK CHECK

Make certain your record-keeping system is working for you. If not, experiment!

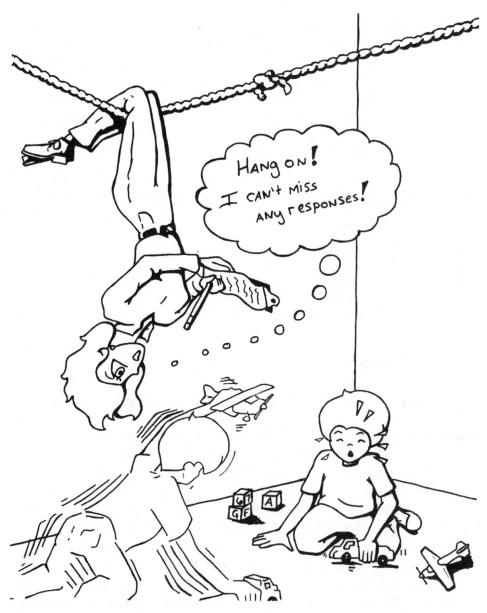

Figure 6–2   At *all* costs.

WAYS TO RECORD

There are many ways to record responses. When a clear-cut response is required (as in objectives 1 and 2 in Exhibit 6–1), a choice of the following notations would be appropriate: 1 (correct) or 0 (incorrect), + (correct) or – (incorrect), √ (correct) or X (incorrect), and Y(es) (correct) or N(o) (incorrect). If the notation is one that may be confusing to your supervisor, a key should be provided on your record sheet in order to avoid misunderstanding. Be consistent, however, with your choice. Use the same notation across clients and over time.

Horizontal versus Vertical Systems

Horizontal record-keeping entails keeping track of responses in a left-to-right sequence going across the page. Vertical record-keeping involves recording responses from top to bottom. A horizontal system is considered "shallow" because less information is obtained. This system usually looks at first attempts only. Second, third, or additional attempts at a stimulus item are not recorded. Adaptations can be made so that horizontal record-keeping can become slightly more effective. Vertical record-keeping is considered a "deep" system in that more information is obtained. It is conducive to recording all attempts made at a stimulus item.

Horizontal Example

In this example, Y(es) will be used to denote a correct response and N(o) will be used to indicate an incorrect response. Twelve responses will be noted in horizontal fashion. They are: **N N Y Y Y N Y Y Y N Y Y.** According to these data, the client responded correctly on 8 of 12 stimulus items, or in 67% of the attempts. On the basis of this data set, it appears that further opportunities were not given to the client to achieve success on the four incorrect stimulus items. If this is the case, this is not good practice, as appropriate techniques should be used to elicit correct responses when the client experiences difficulty. If, however, other opportunities to succeed were given, this system tends to inhibit recording the responses.

The horizontal system can be modified so that each and every response made on a stimulus item is recorded. A response sheet might then contain the following: **NNNYNNYYYNNYYYYYNYYYY.** Most people would interpret these data in the following manner: the client correctly responded on 12 of 20 stimulus items, or on 60% of the attempts. This interpretation is not accurate because there were only 12 stimulus items. The client's performance is misrepresented. Each attempt on a particular stimulus item cannot be weighted equally. That is, a second attempt cannot be counted the same as a first attempt, and a third attempt cannot be counted the same as a second attempt, and so forth. In this example, this faux pas occurred in that all responses were weighted equally. It is not possible to determine at what point one stimulus item ends and the next begins.

A minor modification can be made to rectify this problem. A comma will be added after each stimulus item. In this manner, it is possible to determine the number of attempts before a correct response is attained. Example A is **NNNY, NNY, Y, Y, NNY, Y, Y, Y, NY, Y, Y, Y.** It is now possible to see that there were only 12 original stimulus items. The client correctly responded on 8 of 12 stimulus items, or on 67% of the attempts.

To make an additional point about the inadequacy of a horizontal system, example B is provided. Here, the records on the response sheet are **NNY, NY, Y, Y, NY, Y, Y, Y, NY, Y, Y, Y.** Again, there were 12 stimulus items. The client's performance appears to be the same as that in the last example in that there were correct responses on 8 of the 12 stimulus items (67%). Assuming that the goal was the same and example A was the result from the previous session and example B the result from the present session, it appears that the client did not make progress. This is not the case, however, when second, third, and fourth attempts are considered. In example A, the client correctly responded on 1 of 4 second attempts (25%). In example B, there were correct responses on 3 of 4 second attempts (75%). When third attempts are analyzed, progress is also evident (2 of 3, or 67%, in example A compared with 1 of 1, or 100%, in example B). In example B, fourth attempts were not necessary, although one was needed in example A. With the use of a more thorough analysis, progress was evident.

It is clear that there are problems with any horizontal system. It is now evident why this type of system can be regarded as shallow. The data fall short of that necessary for complete, accurate records. Adaptations can be made to offset, but not eliminate, these inherent problems.

Vertical Example

The same responses to the 12 stimulus items noted in the previous section are again the focus here. This time, however, they will be recorded using a vertical system:

1. **NNY**
2. **NY**
3. **Y**
4. **Y**
5. **NY**

6. **Y**
7. **Y**
8. **Y**
9. **NY**
10. **Y**
11. **Y**
12. **Y**

A quick analysis of the data enables one to determine immediately that the client responded correctly on 8 of 12 items, or in 67% of the attempts. Of the 4 errors, 3 of 4, or 75%, were corrected on the second attempt and 1 additional error was corrected on the third attempt.

With the data set up in the vertical fashion shown, it is easier to scan responses quickly during the therapy session to determine whether a criterion has or has not been met. It is possible to organize the response sheet further to make scanning the data even easier. An example can be found in Exhibit 6–2.

Using this method, data regarding first, second, and third attempts on a stimulus item are readily available. A system like this is more accurate because *all* responses are recorded, and even minimal progress can be detected by analyzing performance on second, third, and further attempts on a stimulus item.

Completed Response Sheet—Vertical System

Let us return to Exhibit 6–2 and see how the response sheet looks when completed. Records of either the client's responses or their outcomes are shown in Exhibit 6–3 using a vertical format.

Please note the responses recorded for objective 3 in Exhibit 6–3. For objectives dealing with the use of language, it is not adequate to note simply whether the client's response was correct or incorrect. If the response was incorrect, it is important to write verbatim what the client said. In this manner, you can analyze the client's errors and use the results of this analysis to determine your therapeutic strategy. The documentation of the client's language can provide justification for continued therapy, progress, and/or carryover. It is also important to indicate the type of cueing used, if any, to help obtain a correct response. In the example given, you can easily see that two of the correct responses were achieved through imitation. It is important to record responses in detail so you have access to this important information.

In summary, clinicians can use either a horizontal system or a vertical system. A horizontal system is not the best approach, even when it is made more useful by

Exhibit 6–2 Sample Response Sheet

	First Attempt	Second Attempt	Third Attempt
1.	N	N	Y
2.	N	Y	
3.	Y		
4.	Y		
5.	N	Y	
6.	Y		
7.	Y		
8.	Y		
9.	N	Y	
10.	Y		
11.	Y		
12.	Y		

making modifications—many of which are borrowed from the vertical system. The vertical system is better for measuring slight improvement. Therefore, the vertical system would be better for you to adopt early in your career.

QUICK CHECK

Whether you are using a horizontal system or a vertical one, make certain you are accounting for the client's repeated attempts on a stimulus item.

ACCOUNTABILITY

Up to now in this chapter we have stressed how accurate records are necessary for effective therapy. Record-keeping has another purpose that needs to be addressed. As in all allied health fields, you must be accountable for the decisions and actions you take in serving each client.

In its most elemental and nonlegal form, accountability is knowing what to do and doing what you know (assuming proficiency in both knowledge and practice and being able to document both). Records document that you knew the problem and provided appropriate services. Without records, or with inadequate records,

Exhibit 6–3 Completed Response Sheet

Objective 1 (Receptive Identification)		Objective 2 (Expressive Identification)	
1. eye	Y	1. eye	NY
2. ear	Y	2. ear	NY
3. knee	NY	3. knee	NNY
4. hand	Y	4. hand	Y
5. foot	NNY	5. foot	NNY
6. mouth	Y	6. mouth	NY
7. elbow	NY	7. elbow	NNY
8. chin	NY	8. chin	NNY
9. face	Y	9. face	Y
10. finger	NY	10. finger	NNY

Objective 3 (Production of Is + Verbing)

1.	dog running	N	dog is run	N	dog is running	I
2.	cat is climb	N	cat climbing	N	cat is climbing	I
3.	boy walking	N	boy is walking	Y		
4.	girl is write	N	girl is writing	Y		
5.	man is driving	Y				
6.	lady is reading	Y				
7.	cow is mooing	N	cow is mooing	Y		
8.	cat is walking	Y				
9.	boy is throwing	Y				
10.	girl is walking	Y				

Note: I = imitation.

other clinicians cannot review your work in preparation for taking on the client and you cannot defend yourself against claims that you acted inappropriately in designing and executing a therapy program. Records are often the only resource to demonstrate that you acted responsibly and that you have fulfilled your obligations to the client, to the profession, and to yourself.

TRACKING CLINICAL HOURS

There is no set number of clinical hours required on the undergraduate level. Individual universities determine the number of clinical hours necessary for their own programs. The American Speech-Language-Hearing Association (ASHA) currently (1997) requires a total of 375 clock hours to be obtained in supervised clinical observation (25 hours) and clinical practicum (350 hours) in order to be eligible to apply for a Certificate of Clinical Competence (CCC) after earning a master's degree. A maximum of 100 hours earned in practicum at the undergraduate level can count toward the hours necessary to obtain this certification. At this time, it is not possible to know *which* 100 hours will be counted; therefore, it is necessary to keep track of *all* possible hours that could conceivably count toward certification. To do this, it is necessary to understand ASHA's observation and clinical practicum requirements. The basic requirements as given in the *Membership & Certification Handbook: Speech-Language Pathology* (ASHA, 1997) are cited to provide direction for pursuing CCC in speech-language pathology. (The author's commentary appears in italics and brackets.) These requirements are as follows:

> Applicants for either Certificate must complete at least 25 clock hours of supervised observation prior to beginning the initial clinical practicum. . . . Those 25 clock hours must concern the evaluation and treatment of children and adults with disorders of speech, language, or hearing. (p. 14)

> No more than 25 of the clock hours may be obtained from participation in staffings in which evaluation, treatment, and/or recommendations are discussed or formulated, with or without the client present. (p. 15) *[Meetings with practicum supervisors may not be counted. Ample opportunity should be available to obtain these hours at the graduate level. Therefore, it is not necessary for undergraduates to track hours in this category.]*

> At least 250 of the 350 clock hours must be completed in the professional area for which the Certificate is sought while the applicant is engaged in graduate study. (p. 15) *[All graduate coursework and graduate clinical practicum hours completed after January 1, 1994, must be started and finished at programs that are accredited by the Council on Academic Accreditation in Audiology and Speech-Language Pathology (CAA).]*

> At least 50 supervised clock hours must be completed in each of three types of clinical setting. (p. 15) *[It is necessary to gain three diverse experiences. Each of these experiences must be unique as determined by your*

*educational program. For example, if you provide services in two differ-
ent rehabilitation hospitals but only receive experience with a stroke
population, these settings would not be considered diverse. On the other
hand, if you service a stroke population in one rehabilitation hospital and
a brain injured population in the other, these would serve as two of the
three required diverse settings.]*

The applicant must have experience in the evaluation and treatment of
children and adults and with a variety of types and severities of disorders
of speech [articulation, fluency, voice, dysphagia], language, and hearing." (p. 15) *[This experience is supposed to include both individual and
group client contact. However, ASHA does not specify the number of
hours specifically needed in either group or individual therapy. Further,
ASHA does not define or clarify "severities." So, to be safe, make certain
that you conduct both individual and group therapy. Also make certain
that the problems of your clients range in severity.]*

At least 250 of the 350 supervised clock hours must be in speech-language pathology. At least 20 of those 250 clock hours must be completed
in each of the eight categories listed below.

1. Evaluation: speech disorders in children
2. Evaluation: speech disorders in adults
3. Evaluation: language disorders in children
4. Evaluation: language disorders in adults
5. Treatment: speech disorders in children
6. Treatment: speech disorders in adults
7. Treatment: language disorders in children
8. Treatment: language disorders in adults (p. 16)

*[Evaluation consists of screening, assessment, and diagnosis accom-
plished before therapy begins. Formal re-evaluations are also included in
the evaluation category. Clock hours devoted to counseling associated
with the evaluation/diagnostic process may be counted. Screening activities cannot comprise the majority of evaluation hours in each category.
Included under treatment is clinical management (both direct and indirect services), progress in monitoring activities, and counseling. On the
undergraduate level, it is best to track only direct clinical services. There
should be ample opportunity to obtain hours in indirect services during
graduate school.]*

Up to 20 clock hours in the major professional area may be in related disorders. . . . Hours may be obtained for activities related to the prevention of communication disorders and the enhancement of speech, language, and communicative effectiveness. Similarly, activities implemented to prevent the onset of speech/language disorders and their causes as well as efforts to advance the development and conservation of optimal communication may be counted. . . . (p. 16) *[Hours earned in graduate school are usually counted in this category. It is not necessary to track these hours on the undergraduate level.]*

At least 35 of the 350 clock hours must be in audiology. At least 15 of those 35 clock hours must involve the evaluation or screening of individuals with hearing disorders, and at least 15 must involve habilitation/rehabilitation of individuals who have hearing impairment. (p. 16)

Palmer and Mormer (1992) have conveniently outlined the clinical observation and clinical practicum requirements in speech-language pathology (Table 6–2). Their chart provides a good summary of ASHA's certification requirements, which were previously presented in this section. Palmer and Mormer said, "This type of chart makes the needed hours apparent and assists in encouraging the students to take responsibility for accurate and precise record keeping" (p. 54). This chart will enable you to see at a glance exactly where you need to obtain hours.

Clinical Hours Tracking Sheets

To have pertinent information regarding clinical requirements at your fingertips, three different forms will now be offered. Using any of these forms will assist with tracking clinical requirements in a painless fashion. The choice of which form to use should be guided by your needs and your personal preference. The first form can be found in Exhibit 6–4.

Another form (Exhibit 6–5) was designed by Palmer and Mormer (1992). They present a paper-and-pencil tracking sheet for use each semester. Hegde and Davis' (1995) form (Exhibit 6–6) will likewise assist you in keeping track of your clinical hours.

You will find one of these forms extremely helpful for recording your clinical practicum contacts, so make the choice, try it, and, if you like it, stick with it. Should you not find it appropriate, switch to another. Be sure to transfer your hours, though.

Table 6–2 Supervised Clinical Observation and Clinical Practicum Requirements in Speech-Language Pathology

	25 c.h.				Clinical Observation
Minimum 375 Clock Hours (c.h.)	Min 350 c.h. Clinical Practicum (Max 25 c.h. Staffings) (Min 50 c.h. in each of three types of clinical settings	Speech-Language—Min 250 c.h.	Min 20		1. Evaluation: Speech disorders in children
			Min 20		2. Evaluation: Speech disorders in adults
			Min 20		3. Evaluation: Language disorders in children
			Min 20		4. Evaluation: Language disorders in adults
			Min 20		5. Treatment: Speech disorders in children
			Min 20		6. Treatment: Speech disorders in adults
			Min 20		7. Treatment: Language disorders in children
			Min 20		8. Treatment: Language disorders in adults
			Max 20		9. Related disorders
		Audiology (Max 100, Min 35)	Min 35	Min 15	Evaluation or screening of individuals with hearing disorders
				Min 15	Habilitation/rehabilitation of individuals who have hearing impairment

Source: Reprinted with permission from C. V. Palmer and E. A. Mormer, Tracking Clinical Learning Experience, *Asha*, August, p. 53 © 1992, American Speech-Language-Hearing Association.

It is recommended that hours be recorded in the appropriate slots on the form at the end of those days on which clients are seen. Assuming that most encounters are in half-hour increments, record 0.5 (half-hour), 1.0 (one hour), 1.5 (one and a half hours) in the appropriate places. Hegde and Davis (1995) recommend use of the following guidelines for reporting fractions of hours: 55 minutes = 0.9, 50 minutes = 0.8, 45 minutes = 0.75, 40 minutes = 0.7, 35 minutes = 0.6, 25 minutes = 0.4, 20 minutes = 0.3, 15 minutes = 0.25, 10 minutes = 0.2, and 5 minutes = 0.1.

Exhibit 6–4 Observation and Practicum Requirements

Observation and Practicum Requirements

NAME: _____ DATES: _____

Clinical Observation
(25 hours)

Evaluation			**Treatment**		
	Children	*Adults*		*Children*	*Adults*
Speech			Speech		
Language			Language		
Hearing			Hearing		

Clinical Settings
(3 types of settings)

1. _____
2. _____
3. _____

Clock Hours
(250 Hours)*

Evaluation			**Treatment**		
	Children	*Adults*		*Children*	*Adults*
Speech			Speech		
Language			Language		

Audiology
(35 Hours)

Evaluation or screening (15 hours)
Habilitation or rehabilitation (15 hours)
*A minimum of 20 hours is necessary in each of the eight slots.

Exhibit 6–5   Student Worksheet for Recording Clinical Practicum Contacts in Speech-Language Pathology

Clinic Practicum Contacts—Speech Language Path.   Student Name:
Student Clinician Record Log   Student ID #:

Date	Client Information		Setting	Contact Hours by Evaluation Type									Init.
	Last name	Age		1	2	3	4	5	6	7	8	9	
	TOTALS:												

Evaluation types: (1) Evaluation: Speech disorders in children, (2) Evaluation: Speech disorders in adults, (3) Evaluation: Language disorders in children, (4) Evaluation: Language disorders in adults, (5) Treatment: Speech disorders in children, (6) Treatment: Speech disorders in adults, (7) Treatment: Language disorders in children, (8) Treatment: Language disorders in adults, (9) Related disorders

Source: Reprinted with permission from C.V. Palmer and E.A. Mormer, Tracking Clinical Learning Experience, *Asha*, August, p. 54, © 1992, American Speech-Language-Hearing Association.

Exhibit 6–6   Worksheet for Recording Clinical Practicum Hours in Speech-Language Pathology

University Speech and Hearing Center

Clinical Practicum Hours

Student   Supervisor   Semester

Practicum Site   Circle one: Adults   Children

EVALUATION/DIAGNOSTIC HOURS							
Date	Language	Articulation	Voice	Fluency	Other	Staffing	Supervisor Initials
Total							

TREATMENT HOURS							
Date	Language	Articulation	Voice	Fluency	Other	Staffing	Supervisor Initials
Total							

Supervisor's signature   License #   ASHA CCC Account #

Source: Reprinted with permission by Singular Publishing Group, Inc. (San Diego, California), M. N. Hegde and D. Davis, *Clinical Methods and Practicum in Speech-Language Pathology*, 2nd ed., p. 310, © 1995.

Use one tracking sheet per week. At the end of the week, compile the data. It is advantageous to make notes on the back such as the client's last name, dates of sessions, and client's problem. At the end of the second week, compile the data from both sheets. At the end of the third week, compile the data from all three sheets, and so on. At the end of the semester, compile all the sheets and then immediately have your form signed by your supervisor. If he or she has any questions regarding your hours at this time, you should be able to find the answers easily by consulting all of your tracking sheets, especially the notes made on the back. Do not throw any tracking sheets away until your supervisor signs the composite tracking sheet covering the entire semester.

QUICK CHECK

Know what ASHA's requirements are. Make certain you meet them!

IMPORTANT ADVICE

There are two pieces of advice that should be followed at the appropriate point in your professional life. The first pertains to clinical hours. Upon completion of any practicum experience, have your immediate supervisor sign an "hours" sheet. Once an "hours" sheet is signed, make two copies. Have the secretary place one in your departmental student file, and you place the other in your own personal professional file.

If the signing of an "hours" sheet is part of the standard operating procedure of your clinical program, make certain the sheet is at least as detailed as one in this book. If it is not as detailed, also use one of the forms presented here and have your supervisor sign both of them. The supervisor's signature verifies that these are the number of hours actually earned within the designated categories. Also obtain your supervisor's ASHA account number because this information will be needed when completing your paperwork for certification. If this advice is not followed, it could be time-consuming to reconstruct this information later. The supervisor may have taken a professional position elsewhere, and it may be difficult to locate him or her to verify practicum hours or to obtain his or her ASHA number. The supervisor may no longer remember you and might not have a record of your clinical hours. Therefore, it is best to have your hour sheet designed as specifically as possible and to have your supervisor sign it in a timely fashion.

The second piece of advice pertains to certification requirements. It is your responsibility to be familiar with ASHA's certification requirements. Read ASHA's current *Membership & Certification Handbook: Speech-Language Pathology* at strategic points throughout your professional schooling. It is suggested that you obtain the most *current* copy of this *Handbook* at three strategic points in your professional career: before your student teaching experience on the undergraduate level, when entering a graduate program, and during the semester preceding graduation. By doing this, you will stay on top of the number of hours needed to meet the certification requirements that are current at that time.

Major changes were made in the certification standards that became effective January 1993. Major changes will probably not occur again for a number of years. Because of the significant impact that certification will have on your professional career, it is extremely important to consult the most **current** *Handbook* to get on the right path and to stay on it so that you meet the clinical practicum requirements for certification.

KNOW IT! USE IT!

After reading this chapter, you should be able to:

1. describe all aspects of the system designed to streamline paperwork
2. state at least eight questions that should be addressed when evaluating your therapy session
3. state four reasons why you might forget to record responses during a session
4. explain a horizontal recording system in detail without error
5. explain a vertical recording system in detail without error
6. state and explain ASHA's certification requirements

REFERENCES

American Speech-Language-Hearing Association. (1997). *Membership & certification handbook: Speech-language pathology.* Rockville, MD: American Speech-Language-Hearing Association.

Hegde, M.N., & Davis, D. (1995). *Clinical methods and practicum in speech-language pathology* (2nd ed.). San Diego, CA: Singular.

Kibbee, R., & Lilly, G. (1989). Outcome-oriented documentation in a psychiatric facility. *Journal of Quality Assurance, 10,* 16.

Leahy, M. (1995). *Disorders of communication: The science of intervention.* London: Whurr Publishers.

Palmer, C., & Mormer, E. (1992). Tracking clinical learning experience. *Asha, 34,* 53–55.

CHAPTER 7

Enhancing Performance

CHAPTER HIGHLIGHTS

- *optimal seating arrangement*
- *correct usage of reinforcement during therapy*
- *use of praise and encouragement during testing*
- *the impact of providing appropriate verbal models*
- *avoiding "smothering the client" and fostering dependency*
- *the importance of choice constancy*
- *rationales for presenting materials in a left-to-right, top-to-bottom sequence*
- *the importance of analyzing elicitation techniques*
- *a hierarchy of articulation cueing techniques*
- *using questions sparingly*
- *avoiding the appearance of being a fool and being overpowering*
- *presenting clear, precise, and concise directions*
- *devising effective receptive tasks*
- *conducting group therapy sessions*
- *a rationale for avoiding habits that may be misinterpreted*
- *a rationale for avoiding game emphasis*
- *appropriate session emphasis*
- *maximizing carryover*
- *using effective sign language instruction*
- *appropriate session opening and closing*

The purpose of this chapter is to provide you with suggestions to make your sessions run more smoothly and to enable you to perform more efficiently and effectively during the therapeutic process. This chapter does not provide general therapeutic techniques or theories because this knowledge should have previously been obtained, although it may be necessary to remind you occasionally of some of this information by providing examples that show how classroom knowledge is incorporated into the therapeutic process. When you complete this chapter, you should be able to deal with many of the common problems experienced as you commence providing clinical services.

PROBLEM AND SOLUTION 1: SEATING ARRANGEMENT

Record-Keeping

Beginning clinicians frequently use suboptimum seating arrangements. Naturally, this would not be an issue if the furniture were nailed to the floor and if you were told where to sit and where to seat your client or clients. However, this is usually not the case. You are usually always responsible for arranging the seating and preparing the room prior to the client's arrival. Although a seemingly simple task, problems with the seating arrangement have often been encountered. Fortunately, solutions are available to alleviate these problems.

The clinician, who is usually right-handed, has a tendency to seat the client on her right. This results in the session's records being kept directly under the client's eyes. This is a constant fascination and distraction to the client. Further, while taking a formal test, the client watches the clinician mark the record sheet. Thus, the client has some knowledge about when he responded correctly and when he did not. This is information to which the client should not have access because it may bias the testing results.

It may appear that a suitable solution is to place the client across from the clinician. This arrangement will rectify the problem just described, but it creates others. It becomes difficult to reach across the table to provide tactile stimulation when, for example, it is necessary for the client to feel the vibration of your vocal cords or your air stream against his hand. Another type of problem resulting from the seating arrangement arises when the clinician (right-handed) has the client sit on her left and then moves her record-keeping sheet to the left. The reason for this action is not really known but probably results from a need to turn and maintain eye contact with the client. This position proves difficult because the clinician must twist and turn to record a response. No wonder clinicians get the impression that record-keeping is bothersome. We all would find it to be so if this were the way it had to be done.

The two problems that result from these seating arrangements can be easily rectified by placing the record-keeping sheet off to the side of the clinician's writing hand. If the clinician is right-handed, records should be kept on the right side. If the clinician is left-handed, records should be kept on the left side. The client

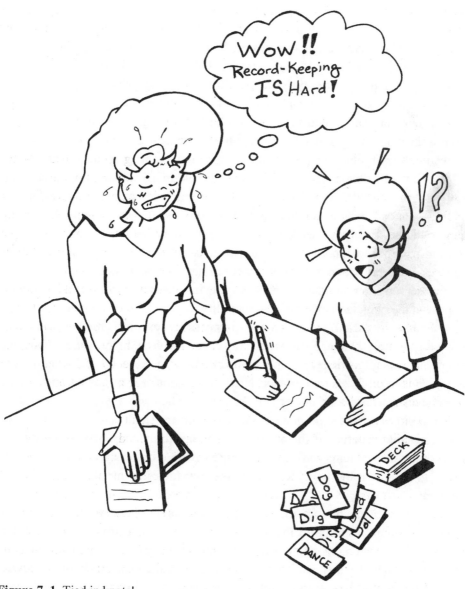

Figure 7–1 Tied in knots!

should be on the side farthest from the clinician's writing hand. For the right-handed clinician, the client should be on the clinician's left. If the clinician is left-handed, the client should be on the clinician's right. These adjustments will minimize the client's distraction by keeping records out of immediate sight and eliminate the clinician's gyrations. These changes should result in smoother-running sessions.

These more effective seating arrangements enable the clinician's dominant hand to be free to keep records while the other hand manipulates the clinical materials (turning pages, flipping cards, and so forth). In this manner, the flow of the session is not interrupted while responses are recorded. Consider the consequences of an alternative approach. During an observation I once made, it was noted that a right-handed clinician had seated the client on her left and had placed her record response sheet on her right. It appeared that this clinician was off to a very good start. Instead of "reserving" her right hand for record-keeping purposes, the clinician selected a card with her left hand, put the pen (held in her right hand) down on the table and proceeded to transfer the card from her left to her right hand. After the client responded, the clinician transferred the card back to her left hand. When this happened, the clinician either forgot to record responses or stopped the flow of the session in order to record. The clinician consistently recorded the client's responses, however, when her pen was held in her dominant hand. Merely holding the pen served as a reminder and played a role in consistent record-keeping, which improved the clinician's overall accountability.

Although other seating arrangements are possible, new problems can be created. Take for example what happens when only chairs are used. In this situation, beginning clinicians get yourselves in positions in which you must balance therapy materials and record sheets on your laps. Now the juggling process begins, and recording responses becomes a circus act. As a rule, whenever anything becomes an effort, it either does not get done or gets done inconsistently—which certainly is not acceptable in terms of the actual therapy, not to mention accountability. To remediate this problem, you can use a lapboard to eliminate the juggling act or resort to sitting on the floor. Recording on your tablet on the floor is a feasible alternative.

In summary, it can now be seen how something as simple as modifying the seating arrangement impacts on therapy. When twisting and turning to record responses is eliminated, the task can be performed more quickly. A more productive session results when the flow is not disrupted. Accountability can be improved. By making minor adjustments in seating arrangements and related aspects, significant improvement can result.

Client Access

The best clinician cannot "help" a client if there is no access to the client. When working with preschool children with behavior problems or adjustment problems

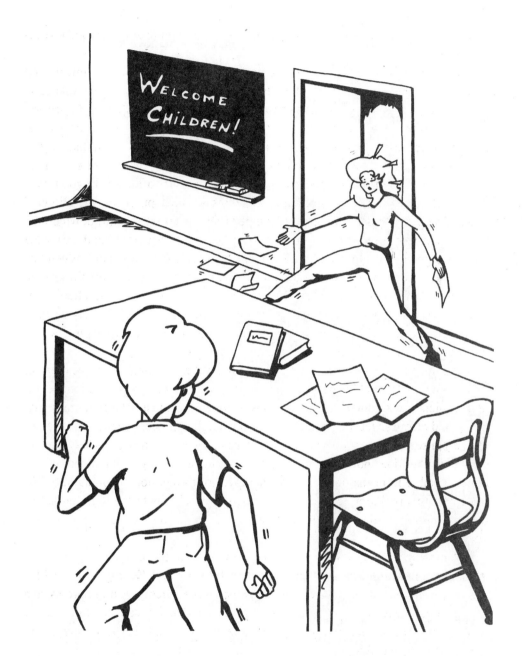

Figure 7–2 Preventing the runaway.

(adjusting to the newness and unfamiliarity of the therapeutic situation and clinician or separating from a significant other), it may be necessary to seat yourself between the child and the door in case "interception" becomes necessary. These children have not yet become acclimated and may try to remove themselves from the new and unfamiliar situation, or they may try to find the familiar person waiting for them by making a dash for the door. If this happens and the child is successful, you will find yourself running down the hall after the child or coaxing the child to return to the therapy room. Because of these interferences, therapy is nonproductive. Less time might be lost if you adhere to the solution of positioning yourself between the child and the door.

QUICK CHECK

Before starting each session, make certain your seating arrangement is efficient for both record-keeping and client access.

PROBLEM AND SOLUTION 2: REINFORCEMENT

For you to be effective during various aspects of the therapeutic process, the theory of reinforcement must be understood and appropriately applied. Non-goal-directed behaviors must not be *accidentally* reinforced, and goal-directed behaviors must not be *inappropriately* reinforced. The manner in which reinforcement is used differs depending on the task. Reinforcement techniques are not the same during therapy and testing.

Therapy

Reinforcement is frequently used during therapy sessions. Properly used, it can be instrumental in establishing and/or maintaining certain behaviors. When reinforcement is not used appropriately, detrimental results can occur. Let us explore this further.

Accidental and Inappropriate Usage

Clinicians have a tendency to use a select word or a few select words when providing verbal reinforcement. The word "good" is frequently chosen to perform this function. Although variety is preferred, there is nothing wrong with using the word "good" during the session if it is only used for the purpose of reinforcement; however, this is usually not the case. This word is also frequently used to convey a casual comment or to serve as a conversational filler.

This example occurred in a session when the goal was to correctly produce the /r/ phoneme in the initial position of words. The clinician's use of "good" as a casual comment followed the client's extraneous response. The client was shown a picture of a robe (which happened to be blue) in an attempt to elicit the word "robe." The following occurred:

Client: I like blue.

Clinician: You like blue? Good.

The clinician's intent was not to reinforce the client but simply to acknowledge his comment. Thus, the word "good," which is used to reinforce session goals should not be used for unrelated purposes because its *reinforcing effect* will be weakened or lost. It is important to note that the same comments would be appropriate if initiating conversation or spontaneously commenting were the goals of the session. Then the clinician's use of "good" would be justified if it immediately followed the client's response. A more appropriate way of dealing with the client's extraneous comment would be to respond briefly to the content. Responses such as "I like blue, too" or "Blue is my favorite color, too" would be appropriate.

Next is an example showing inappropriate usage of "okay" ("OK"). Note what happened in this interaction.

Clinician: (models for client) Say /s/.

Client: (produces a distorted /s/)

Clinician: OK. That wasn't right.

The client was immediately reinforced for producing a distortion of the /s/ phoneme. This unintentional reinforcement occurred when the clinician said "OK" immediately following the client's response. This beginning clinician knew that the client's production was not correct and had no intention of reinforcing this incorrect production. This beginning clinician used "OK" as a filler to give herself an extra moment to think of another therapeutic technique to implement in order for the client to correctly produce the target phoneme. Reinforcement is a powerful tool and must always be used appropriately. When mixed feedback signals are given to the client, correction of the problem will take longer, and frustration (of both the client and beginning clinician) is likely to occur. The best solution to this problem is to decrease overall "OK" usage.

Other, less obvious, examples of inappropriate and accidental reinforcement are presented here. In this example, the beginning clinician was working with a client who was functioning on a low cognitive level. "Mouthing" objects, which is not considered desirable behavior, was characteristic of this client. The clinician gave objects to the client one at a time and said, "What do you do with _____ ?" First, a car was presented. The client immediately put the car in her mouth. The clinician removed the car, said "no" to indicate that the response was not appropriate, and modeled both the correct action as well as suitable language. A ball was then presented. The client again mouthed the ball. The clinician responded in the same manner as just indicated. Next, a cup was presented. The obvious happened: The client mouthed the cup and the clinician reinforced the client for this behavior. In essence, the clinician reinforced the child's undesirable mouthing behavior. It is this same exact behavior that the clinician tried to extinguish in the first two trials that is now being reinforced. In anticipation of the child's extremely predictable response, the clinician should not have presented a mouthing object.

Another example of inappropriate and accidental reinforcement is presented. During a different interaction with different participants, the clinician reminded the client to swallow because one of the goals was to eliminate drooling. At one point in the session, the clinician sat on the floor and placed the client across her lap in a supine position with the client's head tilted posteriorly. After a period, the clinician reinforced the client for not drooling. Reinforcement in this case was not deserved because of the laws of gravity. It would have been impossible to drool in that position. The client should not receive reinforcement under circumstances in which she is not in control of the behavior.

Continuous Reinforcement

It is known that continuous reinforcement is most effective for establishing a new skill or behavior. Initially, each correct response should be reinforced, and this reinforcement should immediately follow the client's correct response. The following excerpt is taken from a session in which correct imitation of the /t/ phoneme in the initial position of words was the goal. Please note that every correct response was immediately reinforced.

Clinician: Say "ten."

Client: Ken.

Clinician: Raise your tongue tip. Say "ten."

Client: Ten.

Clinician: Good! Say "top."

Client: Top.

Clinician: Super! Say "to."

Client: To.

Clinician: Very nice!

Intermittent Reinforcement

Once a new skill is *established,* the reinforcement schedule is changed to an intermittent one. This schedule type reduces the possibility of satiation during therapy and also produces greater resistance to extinction. One type of intermittent reinforcement is called fixed-ratio, and reinforcement occurs after a fixed number of responses. It may occur after every third or fifth response or whatever number is considered appropriate when taking the client, his ability, his needs, and the type of therapy into account. The client's goal in this example is to correctly produce the /p/ phoneme in all positions of words in sentences. The example is:

Client (looking at pictures): The pup is big.

Clinician: This one.

Client: The pot fell.

Clinician: Next!

Client: The pie is good.

Clinician: This one.

Client: The cup broke.

Clinician: Nice work! Keep going!

Client: The cup is colorful.

Client: His name is Pete.

Client: The pan is rusty.

Client: Take a pill.

Clinician: Super! Try some more.

This example shows reinforcement being given after every fourth correct response.

Specific and Varied

Reinforcement should be both specific (directly related) to the task performed and varied. In this manner, the client knows exactly what behavior is being reinforced and does not become bored hearing the clinician say the same thing again and again. In this first set of examples, reinforcement is not specific, nor is it varied. Examples are:

Clinician: Point to *chair.*

Client: (points to *chair*)

Clinician: Good!

———

Clinician: Say /s/.

Client: /s/.

Clinician: Good!

———

Clinician: (trying to elicit regular plural; pointing to picture) One cat, TWO _____. . . .

Clients: . . . . cats.

Clinician: Good!

Notice that in the first set of examples, the clinician's reinforcement consisted solely of usage of the word *good.* It is obvious it was not varied, but, in addition, it was not specific to the task. Reinforcement makes more of an *impact* when one knows why he or she is being reinforced. It also makes more of an impact when the reinforcing words are changed to best fit the client's response.

The second set of examples will demonstrate usage of specific as well as varied reinforcement. These examples are:

Clinician: Point to *chair.*

Client: (points to *chair*)

Clinician: Good pointing!

———

Clinician: Say /s/.

Client: /s/.

Clinician: Great sound!

Clinician: (trying to elicit regular plural; pointing to picture) One cat, TWO _____ . . .

Clients: . . . cats.

Clinician: Super! You said "cats."

Note that in the second set of examples, the clinician's reinforcement was not always the same. It was varied, but, more importantly, it was specific to each task. In this way, the client is reminded of why he was reinforced. Because the reinforcement is varied, the clinician appears to be more involved in the therapy session. You should strive to use both specific and varied reinforcement.

Tangible

Tangible reinforcement should follow the same rules as verbal reinforcement. Goal-directed behaviors should be reinforced. Non–goal-directed behaviors should not be reinforced. An example is given based on a session in which the goals were to correctly produce the /s/ phoneme in isolation and to correctly produce the /l/ phoneme in the initial position of words. At the end of the session, this particular beginning clinician said, "Because you were good, you get a sticker." The implication is that because the client behaved, he earned a sticker. Nowhere in the goals for the session was behavior mentioned. Also, a determination of whether a client behaved requires subjective judgment. The awarding of a sticker was not in any way based on the client's performance on the goals.

For reinforcement to be effective, the client should be aware of his exact requirements at the start of the session. The explanation must be presented in a manner that the client can understand. Some suggestions are:

Clinician: If you get 100 good responses, you can connect the dots from 1 to 30.

Clinician: Every time you produce a good /s/, put a chip in the cup. If the cup is full at the end of the session, you'll earn a sticker.

Clinician: If 90% of your responses are correct, you can color three leaves at the end of the session.

———

Clinician: When you produce a good /l/, cross off one of these balloons. If all the balloons are crossed off at the end of the session, you'll earn a sticker. (The page contained 100 balloons.)

The first and third examples are more complex than the second and fourth. It is important that directions are presented at a level that the client understands. In the event it actually is "behavior" you want to reinforce, it must be stated in a goal. An example is given for a client who interrupts each session by getting out of his chair an average of five times. One must remember that the client cannot be expected to eliminate the disruptive behavior completely as soon as the goal is instituted. Therefore, do not set the goal so high that the client cannot experience success. Also remember that earning a sticker is only rewarding to the client if he wants one. If it is not rewarding, find something that is. An example based on behavior is:

Clinician: Here are four chips (points). Every time you get out of your chair, you'll lose a chip. At the end of the session, if any chips are still here (points), you will earn a sticker. If there are no chips, you will not earn a sticker.

Notice that now the client is made aware of the expectations. He now knows that earning the sticker, connecting the dots, coloring the leaves, and so forth depends on his performance on the goals of the session. He knows exactly what has to be done to earn the tangible reinforcement. A goal should not be set so high that the client becomes discouraged or so low that the client reaches it long before the session is over. Consult your records regarding the client's performance from the last session to help establish realistic expectations for the next session.

Naturalistic versus Artificial

Naturalistic reinforcement is powerful. This type of reinforcement is concrete and therefore is best used, when possible, with young children or those functioning on a low cognitive level. Naturalistic reinforcement normally occurs in the environment and may include common events such as gaining and sustaining an adult's attention, getting desires and needs met, and engaging in pleasurable human interaction (Reed, 1994). The problem with this type of reinforcement is that it is not used when it can and should be used. For example, let's look at an 18-month-old client who does not use words spontaneously. The client's goal for this session is to imitate names of things that are functional to him. Here is an excerpt from this therapy session showing usage of artificial reinforcers instead of naturalistic re-inforcers.

Clinician: (shows a cookie). Cookie, cookie.

Client: /ʊ/.

Clinician: (knowing the client can get a better approximation) Say "cookie."

Client: /ʊi/.

Clinician: Nice talking!

———

Clinician: (shows the child a jar of bubbles) Bubble, bubble.

Client: /ʌbl̩/.

Clinician: Super!

———

Clinician: (shows client a jar of juice and pours a small amount of juice into a cup. Holds cup toward child). Juice, juice.

Client: /u/.

Clinician: Good talking!

Note that the use of verbal praise in these examples is not going to make much of an impact on this child. Substituting clapping, hugging, dispensing tokens, and so on in this scenario will again result in reinforcement that is artificial. The use of these artificial reinforcers will not teach the client the "power of communication." It will not teach the client that he can manipulate his environment by talking. On the other hand, the client will learn the "power of communication" and that he can manipulate the environment when reinforced in a naturalistic manner. Examples showing usage of natural reinforcement follow:

Clinician: (shows a cookie). Cookie, cookie.

Client: /ʊ/.

>wing the client can get a better approximation) Say
ʊʊokie."

Client: /ʊi/.

Clinician: (gives the child a piece of the cookie to eat)

Client: (the client eagerly eats the cookie piece)

———

Clinician: (shows the child a jar of bubbles) Bubble, bubble.

Client: /ʌbl̩/.

Clinician: (blows bubbles)

Client: (client squeals in delight and "pops" bubbles)

Clinician: (shows client a jar of juice and pours a small amount of
juice into a cup. Holds cup toward child). Juice, juice.

Client: /u/.

Clinician: (extends the cup toward the client)

Client: (takes the cup and drinks the juice)

Naturalistic reinforcers make the most impact when trying to establish behaviors. In addition, they tend to facilitate generalization. It is important to use this type of reinforcement whenever possible. It certainly makes more sense, as the effects are far reaching.

Testing

Reinforcement given during formal testing differs from that given during therapy. Because the purpose behind both of these professional tasks differs, it follows that reinforcement procedures should also differ. The overall goal of therapy is to enable the client to succeed. Initially, the client becomes aware of his success through the clinician's specific feedback for correct responses. Given specific feedback, the client either repeats or changes his response.

The purpose of the testing situation is to determine how the client is currently functioning. Unlike therapy, the client should not be made aware of the correctness or incorrectness of any response, nor should techniques be used to enable the client to produce a better response. Therefore, reinforcement should not be contingent on the correctness of the response but instead should reflect the fact that the client is *performing* the task.

Perhaps it may be more accurate and specific to refer to the terms *praise* and *encouragement* instead of *reinforcement*. Words of praise and/or encouragement are not necessary after each response but should be provided as needed. During the evaluation process, many supervised beginning clinicians have been observed using the extremes of praise and/or encouragement. In one instance, a beginning clinician was observed administering the **Test of Auditory Comprehension of Language** (101 items) without providing any praise and/or encouragement. When questioned about this, she responded that she was not supposed to reinforce the client during testing. At the other extreme, another beginning clinician was observed saying "good" after each of the 101 items. When questioned, this clinician responded that she thought each response had to be reinforced. Note how easily information can be taken out of context and inappropriately applied.

An example portraying correct usage of praise and/or encouragement during administration of the **Peabody Picture Vocabulary Test-III** is given in the following:

Clinician: Show me "bus."

Client: (points to correct response)

Clinician: Show me "drinking."

Client: (points to correct response)

Clinician: Show me "hand."

Client: (points to correct response)

Clinician: Show me "climbing."

Client: (points to correct response)

Clinician: You're working hard! Show me "key."

Client: (points to correct response)

Clinician: Show me "reading."

Client: (points to correct response)

Clinician: Show me "closet."

Client: (points to correct response)

Clinician: Show me "jumping."

Client: (points to incorrect response)

Clinician: You're looking at all the pictures. Show me "lamp."

This example shows praise and encouragement given whenever the clinician believes it is necessary. The particular response provided is not contingent on the correctness of the response but instead is given to the client for performing the task, which, in this case, is pointing. It is important to keep this in mind to prevent the invalidation of results.

QUICK CHECK

Ask yourself whether you are using reinforcement appropriate to the nature of the task. Is it specific and varied? Are you using naturalistic reinforcement when possible?

PROBLEM AND SOLUTION 3: VERBAL MODELS

Because our profession emphasizes speech, language, and communication, it stands to reason that all persons preparing to become clinicians should demonstrate skills in these areas. This is not always the case. Behaviors that do not provide good models need to be eliminated soon after they are identified.

The "OK" Syndrome

Before getting involved in clinical supervision, this author would never have believed that a section of this nature would be necessary in a book intended for students beginning clinical practicum. However, the overuse of "OK" or the "OK syndrome" is abundantly evident during many therapy sessions of beginning clinicians.

Beginning clinicians appear to use "OK" to serve five functions. The first function is using "OK" as a conversational filler. In this instance, "OK" is said for no apparent reason throughout the session. Beginning clinicians do not seem comfortable with pauses or silence occurring within a session. When these moments occur, there is a tendency to interject "OK" although it serves no apparent purpose.

A second usage of "OK" functions as a tag question. In this manner, a statement is made into a nonauthoritative request. An example is:

Clinician: Say it again, *OK*?

A third function of "OK" is that of providing feedback. Often, beginning clinicians do not directly distinguish between correct or incorrect responses. "OK" is said after an incorrect response instead of providing specific feedback. For instance,

Clinician: Say /s/.

Client: /θ/.

Clinician: OK. This time, close your teeth. Say /s/.

A tendency also exists to use "OK" as a positive reinforcer, a fourth function. After a client gives a correct response, "OK" is said. When used in this manner, the clinician is not making a firm commitment to the client's response.

Clinician: Say /s/.

Client: /s/.

Clinician: OK. Say it again.

Note that using "OK" as a positive reinforcer is too vague. Stronger reinforcing words, such as "Great sound!" and "Super /s/!" should be used. They will make more of an impact on the client, and the client will strive harder to achieve that good production consistently.

The last function of "OK" to be addressed is that of answering questions. This, in itself, is not atypical. The manner in which it has been used during therapy is different, however, in that it immediately follows the clinician's use of "OK" as a tag question. In other words, the clinician responds to her own question. An example is:

Clinician: Let's work on /tʃ/, OK? OK.

Overusing any particular word is monotonous for the listener. Because it does not contribute to providing good language and communication models, excessive usage of "OK" should be eliminated.

Breaking the "OK" Habit

Breaking the habit of overusing "OK" is easier said than done. The initial response is disbelief when you are informed that "OK" was used, for example, 22 times in 3 minutes. Until it is brought to your attention and you are aware of the frequency with which you use "OK," it is not possible to understand the need for elimination.

The first step then is to become aware of overusing "OK." Rather than relying on the supervisor's constant reminder, you must recognize and accept responsibility for your frequent usage. This can be done by taping a session (an audiotape is adequate for this purpose) and recording the number of "OKs" used, as well as timing the number of minutes you were involved in speaking. Then, the number of "OKs" used per minute should be calculated. Review the tape and write down the context in which all usages occurred. Analyze why each instance occurred and determine its function. The five functions presented previously can serve as the framework for this analysis. If an "OK" does not fit this framework, place it in an "other" category. Then further analyze all occurrences in this category and determine whether any additional functions can be identified. Once you are aware of your increased usage, you will start to catch yourself as you say "OK," which is the second step to breaking this habit. Soon thereafter, you will move to the third step, which signifies a higher level. In this step, you will be aware that you are about to say "OK." Instead of saying "OK," however, you will quickly shift to either saying something more appropriate or remaining silent. It is in this manner that the "OK" habit will be broken.

Unnatural Production

Beginning clinicians often use unnatural presentation of words for clients to imitate or receptively identify pictures or objects. Emphasis or overexaggeration may be used unconsciously to help the client achieve success. Rather than making the task easier for the client, the task is complicated because words are presented in an unnatural and incorrect manner. For example, one beginning clinician pronounced the word "button" as /'bʌt 'tən/ instead of using the more frequent productions of /'bʌtn̩/ or /'bʌʔn̩/. Her pronunciation was both unnatural and incorrect in that /t/ should only arrest the first syllable and not also release the second syllable. In addition, both syllables were stressed equally instead of only the first syllable receiving primary emphasis. Owing to the unnaturalness of this production, the word takes longer to say, as a deliberate effort must be made. A similar example was found with the word "eating." This beginning clinician pronounced it as /'it 'tɪŋ/ instead of /'it ɪŋ/. Again, the /t/ phoneme should serve only to arrest the first syllable and not also release the second syllable. Once again, this clinician incorrectly placed equal emphasis on both syllables. "Letter" was also incorrectly pronounced. She said /'lɛt 'tɚ/. The same problem discussed with regard to the first two examples is likewise evident. In the word "letter," however, the /t/ phoneme is actually heard as /d/. Therefore, it should be presented phonemically as /lɛd ɚ/.

Instances of unnatural production seem to occur when the emphasis is placed on an individual word or when a word is pronounced out of the context of running speech. It is not possible to present clients with correct and accurate models if words are spoken in an unnatural and incorrect manner. It is essential that words, regardless of the situation, be presented naturally.

Ungrammatical Utterances

It is also important for you to both use and model grammatical utterances. Simply put, if you do not "practice what you preach," respect will be lost and an unfavorable impression may be formed by those observing you. A few frequent examples of ungrammatical usage are "You listened good," "Listen close," and "You're pointing so nice today." Corrections are "You listened well," "Listen closely," and "You're pointing so nicely today."

You need to model utterances when those initiated by a client are not grammatically correct, even if they do not fall under the jurisdiction of a therapeutic objective. This modeling should be done consistently and in a noncondescending manner. For example, if the client says "How much do I got?" the clinician should casually say, "How much do you have? You have. . . ." If the client says "What that is in there?" the clinician should say, "What is that in there? It's a. . . ." If the client says "If it ain't. . . ." the clinician should model, "If it isn't. . . ." The point is that ungrammatical utterances should not be overlooked, nor should the client receive ridicule, reinforcement, or punishment for this usage. Casually state the client's utterance in a corrected fashion and then respond to the client's question or statement.

> ### QUICK CHECK
>
> Audiotape one of your sessions (with permission, of course). Listen to your verbal models. Make certain you are not guilty of using the "OK" syndrome, unnatural production, or ungrammatical utterances.

PROBLEM AND SOLUTION 4: LOQUACIOUSNESS

Loquaciousness refers to excessive talking on your part. Constantly talking is problematic because when you are talking, the client is *not* responding. The client is also not working toward the goal(s) of the session and, consequently, not correcting his problem. Therefore, your loquaciousness has far-reaching effects. The logical solution is for you to stay focused on the goal(s) of the session. Make certain that all of your talking is necessary and relevant (i.e., giving directions, modeling, giving feedback, providing reinforcement, and so forth).

> **QUICK CHECK**
>
> Audiotaping a session (with permission) will again be helpful. Listen to the tape and determine whether all your talking is necessary and relevant.

PROBLEM AND SOLUTION 5: SMOTHERING THE CLIENT

"Smothering the client" refers to the presentation of language beyond the client's expressive linguistic ability. The following occurrence was noted during an observation of a client who was not yet producing single words. A doll fell off the table. The beginning clinician modeled, "The doll fell off the table." This clinician was modeling language that was far beyond the client's linguistic ability. Modeling is more effective when it is either at a level commensurate with, or only a step or two above, the client's current linguistic ability pending the situation. A more effective way to model in this situation is to provide the single word "doll" (while pointing to the object) and then "fall" (while gesturing or re-enacting the action). This could then be followed by production of the two-word utterance "doll fall." Longer or more complex utterances should not be presented because this client is not yet producing single words.

> **QUICK CHECK**
>
> When working with clients having expressive language problems, analyze your language. Make certain you are modeling language either at a level commensurate with, or a step or two above, the client's current linguistic ability pending the situation. Do not model way beyond the client's level!

PROBLEM AND SOLUTION 6: FOSTERING DEPENDENCY

It seems that speech-language pathologists who promote independence are able to legitimately discharge their clients faster than their counterparts who encourage dependency. Successful clinicians encourage their clients to take responsibility for both their problem and their therapeutic program. Leahy (1995) states "experience has shown that successful speakers are those able to take over their own therapy" (p. 225). A logical question to ask at this point is "Who would ever encourage dependency?" However, as one reads on, a clear answer emerges. Dependency is unconsciously encouraged in verbal interaction. Some clinicians subconsciously foster the client's dependency by sharing the client's problem and behaviors, by encouraging the client to perform tasks for the benefit of the clinician and not for his own betterment, and by being authoritarian. According to Leahy (1995), "Therapy which is ever dependent on the clinician is of limited or no value" (p. 225).

A few examples of sharing the problem and behaviors are as follows: "Keep <u>our</u> hands out of <u>our</u> mouth," and "We're going to start <u>our</u> lesson now." One must remember that they are the client's hands, the client's mouth, and the client's lesson. The client should take responsibility for his problem and for his behavior, but this cannot be done unless the clinician gradually relinquishes "control." Examples of encouraging the client to perform tasks for the benefit of the clinician are as follows: "Say it <u>for me</u>," "Read them again <u>for me</u>," and "Can you read this aloud <u>for me,</u> Bill?" The client should be performing the tasks out of his desire to correct his problem and not out of desire to please the clinician. Examples depicting an authoritarian role are as follows: "<u>I</u> want <u>you</u> to listen to me." "<u>I</u> want <u>you</u> to get the ball and the car," and "<u>I</u> want <u>you</u> to get the baby." The intent of these utterances could have been easily conveyed without indirect reference to the power structure as indicated in these examples through usage of *I, you,* and *me.* Revised examples without reference to power structure are "Listen!" "Get the ball and the car!" and "Get the baby!" Furthermore, instructions given in this fashion are simpler and thus will be easier for clients to process and understand.

QUICK CHECK

Analyze your interaction with your clients. Are you encouraging independence or dependency?

PROBLEM AND SOLUTION 7: CHOICE CONSTANCY

When a receptive task involving pictures or objects is presented, it is extremely important to keep the number of choices (the field) constant. The following occurred when observing a beginning clinician working on increasing receptive vocabulary with a client. This clinician placed four pictures on the table (cookie, milk, car, and ball). In this example, the child always responded correctly and the schedule of reinforcement was intermittent. Here is what ensued:

Clinician: Car. Where's the car?

Client: (points to the car)

Clinician: (removes car picture) Cookie. Where's the cookie?

Client: (points to the cookie)

Clinician: (removes cookie picture) Milk. Where's the milk?

Client: (points to the milk)

Clinician: Nice work!

Here is what should have been done.

Clinician: Car. Where's the car?

Client: (points to the car)

Clinician: (removes the picture of the car and adds another picture, perhaps dog) Cookie. Where's the cookie?

Client: (points to cookie)

Clinician: (removes the picture of the cookie and adds another picture, perhaps juice) Dog. Where's the dog?

Client: (points to dog)

Clinician: Great job! (removes the picture of the dog and adds another appropriate picture)

It is hoped that the difference between the examples is obvious. In the first example, the probability of obtaining correct responses increases rather than remains constant. When the client is asked to identify the first picture, a 25% (1 of 4) probability exists that he can respond correctly by chance. When asked to identify the second picture, the probability increases to 33% (1 of 3) and then to 50% (1 of 2) because only two pictures remained. Note that each successive identification became easier for the client as the number of choices decreased.

The chance of randomly getting correct responses remains the same throughout the second example. The client is always presented with a field of four pictures and four novel choices. Thus, the probability of responding correctly remains 25% (1 of 4) throughout the task. Therefore, it is extremely important to replace each selected item with a new item so that the difficulty level remains constant.

The same problem exists when you do not remove each previously selected item. Although the number of pictures remains constant, the number of choices available to the client does not. If a client correctly pointed to one picture, he will not point to that picture again. Thus, the field has decreased as demonstrated in the first example, and the chance factor does not remain constant.

QUICK CHECK

When presenting receptive tasks to a client, answer this question: Am I keeping the number of choices constant?

PROBLEM AND SOLUTION 8: READING SEQUENCE

It is very important to teach a young child skills necessary for the future. To do so, it is necessary to take a young child's native language into account. Look at the language that the child will learn to read. For example, young clients who will be reading English must learn the left-to-right, top-to-bottom sequence. Therefore, it is important that clinicians not present stimuli in an opposing sequence for these future readers of English.

Beginning clinicians have been observed placing stimulus pictures in a bottom-to-top, right-to-left sequence when sitting opposite the young client. There is a tendency to place the material in correct sequence from one's own perspective, but it is important to remember that the client's perspective is reversed. For the English-speaking child, materials should be placed from the child's left to right and from top to bottom. Once you become aware of any violation of this sequence, it is easy to correct.

QUICK CHECK

When placing stimulus materials in front of an English-speaking child, place them from his left to right and from top to bottom.

PROBLEM AND SOLUTION 9: ELICITATION TECHNIQUES

Language

It is extremely important to use techniques that will elicit the desired or target structure. You must strategically design or structure tasks so that the desired response is likely to be obtained. Let us look at some tasks structured by beginning clinicians. In the first example, the beginning clinician is trying to elicit the pronoun "he" as the overall goal is to correctly use the pronouns "he" and "she." Here is an excerpt:

Clinician: (shows a picture) What did the boy drop?

Client: A cookie.

Clinician: Oh, use your special word.

The client's response was perfectly normal and appropriate to this situation. This response was not reinforced, however, because it was not what the beginning clinician wanted to hear. She wanted the client to say "He dropped a cookie," which would be reinforced because the pronoun "he" would be used correctly. In reality, this response is extremely abnormal. First, "normal" children and adults would not answer this question by using a complete sentence. Second, a pronoun is a word that takes the place of a noun or any word used as a noun. "Normal" speakers do not use pronouns until the noun referent is established. Note that this clinician is requiring the client to use pronouns without first establishing the noun referent.

Whenever the target or expected response is not elicited, you should critically evaluate the task. Concentrate on restructuring the task rather than "teaching" the client to be an abnormal communicator, which is, in essence, what happened in the last excerpt.

Possible tasks that are more conducive to eliciting production of "he" or "she" should be implemented. Have the client tell you about Billy (his best friend). The client will use the proper noun "Billy" once or twice, but then should substitute the proper noun with the pronoun "he." If he does not do this spontaneously, provide a model. Another possible task is to give the client two puppets, Tony and Annie. With the help of the puppets, the client is supposed to build a structure (bridge, house, and so forth) with blocks. The building is to be done behind a screen, and the client is supposed to explain how Tony and Annie are building their structure. The screen is essential, as the client will have to be more verbal and descriptive because you will not have access to the information through the visual modality. If the client does not spontaneously start using the appropriate pronouns after a few references to the nouns, start modeling.

The two suggestions just given are conducive to pronoun elicitation. Modifications will be made if the client confuses the two pronouns. Two main points should be remembered. You should always carefully design the task so that the target behavior is elicited, and you should also be certain that normal communication is emphasized.

Here are some additional examples. The target response in the first excerpt is usage of the regular past tense. It is present progressive tense in the latter excerpt. Although the target structure differs in the two examples, the same points are evident.

Clinician: (rolls a ball across the room) What rolled?

Client: The ball.

Clinician: Say the whole thing.

———

Clinician: (shows a picture) What is the girl doing?

Client: Jumping.

Clinician: Say the whole thing.

It is hoped that it is now realized that both of the client's responses are correct and appropriate. The reason that the target responses were not produced is because the tasks were not properly designed to elicit them. The tasks as designed are conducive to elicit either a Noun or an Article + Noun response in the first example and a Verb + ing response in the second example. The responses are not conducive to usage of the regular past or present progressive tenses. Therefore, the client should not be penalized when, in fact, he is performing correctly and in a normal manner. If one has to give the client instructions such as "use your special word" or "say the whole thing," the task needs to be redesigned. In most cases, it is your stimulus that is problematic and not the client's response.

Articulation

Beginning clinicians have frequently been observed trying to elicit correct production of errored phonemes. Often you are not adept at using cueing and prompting or presenting cues and prompts in any logical order. A hierarchy of cues and prompts are presented here, ranging from those providing the maximum amount of support to those providing the least amount. Bain (1994) provides eight cues that can be used to help a client produce an errored sound correctly. Each cue is stated, summarized, and elaborated as follows:

1. **Manipulation of articulators.** When a child has difficulty producing a phoneme, it is often necessary to manipulate the articulators. For example, when attempting production of an /s/ phoneme with a client who constantly produces θ/s, it may be necessary to use a tongue depressor to push the tongue behind the teeth so that an acceptable production is possible. Another example focuses on production of /p/. When the client produces /p/ labiodentally, it may be necessary to place your thumb on the client's lower lip and index finger of the same hand on the upper lip in order to get the client's lips to come together while also preventing the upper teeth from getting involved in the production.

2. **Placement cues.** This cue is frequently referred to as "phonetic placement." You describe and/or demonstrate the position of the articulators for production of a particular phoneme. For example, if a client frequently produces θ/s, provide the following phonetic placement cue: "Put your teeth together."

3. **Visual and tactile imagery.** This particular type of cueing can also help clients produce errored phonemes correctly. Bain's example is "if a child stops fricatives, says /t/ for /s/, the clinician could talk about dripping versus flowing sounds, or run a finger down the child's arm to represent frication and tap the child's arm to represent stops in order to facilitate correct production" (1994, p. 18).

4. **Prosodic emphasis.** Vary the amount of emphasis placed on the target sound by increasing the intensity and duration. For example, if the error sound is /s/ in the word /sʌn/, it could be presented to the child by "Say /ssssssʌn/." This unnatural emphasis would, however, be eliminated as soon as the client was capable of correct production.

5. **Frequency of stimulus presentation.** Determine the number of times a stimulus is presented prior to requesting the client to respond. You can choose to produce the target phoneme five times slowly and distinctly before expecting the client to respond. There should be silence between your productions and the client's response in order to maximize concentration.

6. **Model of presentation.** You can choose to present an auditory model alone. An example is "Listen. Say /s/." If this is the model presented, the client is only listening to you but not watching. You can also decide to present an auditory and visual model such as "Watch. Listen. Say /s/." In this latter example, the client should be watching as well as listening to you. Obviously, the use of both modalities (visual and auditory) gives the client more support than using any single modality alone.

7. **Phonetic context.** The context in which a phoneme occurs influences production. Some phonemes surrounding an errored phoneme may serve to facilitate pro-

duction. It is known that /t/ preceding /s/ helps many clients achieve correct production. Examples are *cats, boats, boots,* and so on. As Bain (1994) mentions, "the **Deep Test of Articulation** (McDonald 1964) is a useful tool for identifying the influence of surrounding sounds on an errored sound" (p. 17).

8. **Contrasts—minimal pairs.** A client's productions of sounds seems to be influenced by presenting stimulus materials that contrast the errored phoneme with the target phoneme. Present two pictures, each depicting one word of the minimal pair. One picture will contain the target phoneme, and the other will contain the client's usual misarticulated phoneme. A minimal pair that can be used for the process of stopping is "toe" and "sew."

QUICK CHECK

The type of cue or prompt that should be used with a particular client depends totally on the client. Start at the point at which the client is likely to have success. If the client never correctly produces the phoneme, begin with the prompt or cue that will give the maximum amount of help or provide the most support. In this case, *manipulation of articulators* would be a logical starting point if the target phoneme is one that can be approached in this manner. If *manipulation of articulators* cannot be used for a particular target phoneme, try another prompt or cue such as a *placement cue,* which still provides a lot of support.

On the other hand, if the child is able to correctly produce the target phoneme using cues or prompts providing maximum success, continue decreasing the amount of support. Provide prompts or cues that gradually decrease the amount of support in order to enable the client to correctly produce the target phoneme spontaneously.

PROBLEM AND SOLUTION 10: USE QUESTIONS SPARINGLY

A good rule of thumb is never ask a client a question when you will not accept the response. Beginning clinicians have a tendency to start sessions on the wrong foot. An example is as follows:

Clinician: Do you want to look at these pictures?

Client: No!

Now what are you going to do? Those of you who have been observed under these circumstances end up giving the client 10 different reasons why he has to look at the pictures and then arguing results. Note that the whole situation could be avoided if the session were started differently. An example is:

Clinician: Pick a card. Remember to use a good sound.

Now the client is not given the opportunity to say "no." As a result, you do not have to take valuable time away from the session to provide a lengthy explanation or to argue. The implication is not that clients will never refuse to perform a task but that the opportunity to do so should not be initiated by you.

The client should have some control over the session. He should be allowed to make some decisions and choices regarding his therapy sessions, but only when there is no interference with accomplishing goals. Examples are:

Clinician: Should we sit on the floor or at the table?

———

Clinician: Which do you want to do first—the book or the cards?

In the first example, where one sits for therapy has nothing to do with accomplishing goals. Therefore, there will not be any negative consequences. (Keep in mind our discussions of record-keeping in chapter 6.) In the second example, the implication is that the client will "do" both the book and the cards. His decision solely determines the order.

These latter examples differ from the initial one in that the client's responses do not interfere or prevent goal attainment. Other than the actual focus of the therapy session, most clients are capable of making decisions similar to these.

> **QUICK CHECK**
>
> Analyze your use of questions during a session. Never ask a question when you will not abide by the client's response.

PROBLEM AND SOLUTION 11: DO NOT APPEAR TO BE A FOOL

This idea comes from the work of Jon Miller (1981). One of his suggestions for conversations with children is, "Do not play the fool" (p. 12). You are not supposed to ask questions that the child knows you know the answer to because this sets you up as looking like a fool. If you know the answer, you must think that the client does not and that is why the question is asked. If the question is obvious and/or simple, which describes most questions asked during a therapy session, the client feels foolish. Some examples are:

Clinician: What color is this?

Client: Red.

———

Clinician: What is the boy doing?

Client: Running.

———

Clinician: What is this?

Client: Soap.

In these examples, the client knows that you know that the color of the ball is red, that the boy is running, and that the object depicted in the picture is a bar of soap. Because the client knows that you know the "answers," it appears that you think the client does not know this very simple, basic, obvious information. It is perceived as you playing the part of a fool, and it is not appreciated. Although these types of questions are plentiful in formal tests, they can be prevented, with conscious effort, in therapeutic sessions. You will have to abandon your simplistic ways of obtaining responses and be more creative in eliciting these target responses from clients.

Perhaps an alternative to the first example could be accomplished in the context of an activity that the client enjoys. This particular client enjoys building with blocks. If the objective is to have the client indicate the color of objects, the clinician could serve as the "block keeper."

Clinician: (places the container of blocks on her lap) What block do you want?

Client: Red.

Clinician: (holds up a red block) Is this red?

Client: Yes.

Clinician: (hands red block to client)

The second example can be restructured in this manner. The clinician has pairs of action cards. Some things depicted are a boy running, a baby crying, a man reading, a lady sitting, a boy playing, a baby falling, a man sawing, a lady reading, and so forth. The client and clinician are playing "Go Fish." Neither can see the other's cards. The clinician will begin in order to establish the pattern.

Clinician: Find "the baby is crying."

Client: I can't. Go fish! Find "the boy is playing."

Clinician: I can't. Go fish! Find "the man is sawing."

Client: I can't. Go fish! Find "the lady is sitting."

Clinician: Here it is.

Client: I have a match. I get another turn. Find "the man is read-
            ing."

The third example can also be restructured. If the goal is to increase the child's expressive vocabulary, it can be accomplished in this manner. The clinician has a "mystery" box or a "surprise" box filled with specific objects. She shakes it to evoke interest. Once again, the clinician begins in order to establish the pattern.

Clinician: I close my eyes, reach in, and find money.

Client: I close my eyes, reach in, and find soap.

This latter example can be modified if the client is not capable of this linguistic length or complexity.

After analyzing the two sets of examples, you will see that the same responses are being elicited. It is the manner of elicitation that makes the difference. Most clients will not think that anyone is playing the part of a "fool" in the second set of examples.

In order not to be misleading, it is important to note that there may be times when the initial examples presented earlier in this section are appropriate. Appropriateness depends on the client, the client's age, the goals of the session, and the client's level of performance. If your tasks make you or the client feel or appear foolish, then change is necessary.

QUICK CHECK

If your questions can be perceived as simple or obvious by the client, restructuring is necessary. Change the manner of your elicitation.

PROBLEM AND SOLUTION 12: AVOID BEING OVERPOWERING

It is important to make the client feel comfortable in the therapeutic setting.

Although you may be well aware of creating a comfortable and positive clinical environment, you may still overpower your clients, especially children, without being aware of doing so. For example, a form of overpowering occurs when you sit in a big chair and the client sits in a little chair. It also occurs when a child sits on the floor and you either sit on a chair or kneel. In these examples, you "tower" over the client, which serves to magnify your superiority or authority. Establishing authority of this sort is not conducive to creating a comfortable, positive clinical relationship. With some clients, overpowering may be needed. For most clients, it is not!

Overpowering can be prevented in a very simple fashion when you are aware that it is occurring. Eye-to-eye contact is best for all relationships, and a clinical relationship is no different. Being on eye level with the client will minimize a sense of superiority or authority. When the client is a child, minor modifications are necessary. When seated in chairs, this author always lets the child sit on a big chair while sitting on a little chair herself. When the child is on the floor, this author tries to get as low as possible and usually ends up conducting therapy in a prone position. There have also been times when the child sat in a child-sized chair and this author sat on the floor in front of the child. The end result in each of these scenarios is that the client and the clinician are at eye level. In this manner, no one "towers" over the other, and the child should not feel intimidated or overpowered.

QUICK CHECK

Think about how you can overpower a client. Are you guilty?

PROBLEM AND SOLUTION 13: DIRECTIONS

Beginning clinicians have a tendency to use lengthy directions. Lengthy directions tend to confuse the client. They are also time consuming. An example is:

Clinician: If I would say cat, which one would you point to?

It makes more sense to always present clear, precise, and concise directions. Examples of how to reword the direction just presented are:

Clinician: Point to cat!

———

Clinician: Show me cat!

If the client is working on such a basic receptive level, it is possible that an auditory comprehension problem is present. Therefore, the client may experience more success if all stimuli are presented in a less complex fashion.

Another problem that exists with directions is that many beginning clinicians have a tendency to overexplain. An example is:

Clinician: Let's look at these pictures. Look at each picture carefully. Pick out the other member of the pair presented. For example, if I say "cat," point to "dog." If I say "salt," point to "pepper." These types of words are called opposites.

The clinician is overexplaining. She must learn to "get to the point." A revision of the example is as follows:

Clinician: Look at these pictures of opposites. The opposite of "cat" is "dog." Point to "dog." Let's try one. "Up."

QUICK CHECK

Audiotape a session after obtaining appropriate permission. Analyze your directions. Are they clear, precise, and concise?

PROBLEM AND SOLUTION 14: RECEPTIVE TASKS

It is extremely important to make certain that receptive tasks measure exactly what they were designed to measure. In other words, if the client correctly responds, it should be because he understands that which is being assessed. Let us look at this clinician-devised task in which the goal was receptive identification of verbs.

Clinician: (shows the client two pictures. In one, a boy is playing. In the other, the girl is cooking.) Show me "The boy is playing."

Client: (points to the correct picture)

Clinician: Good work!

Although the client correctly responded, he cannot be credited with understanding the verb "play." There is another strategy that the client could have used to respond correctly that has nothing to do with understanding the verb "play." The client could have responded to the noun "boy." Because one picture depicts a boy and the other a girl, understanding of verbs does not even have to be considered when making the choice.

It is obvious that this task has to be changed in order to be effective. Some suggestions are:

> Clinician: (shows the client two pictures. In one, a boy is playing. In the other, a boy is cooking.) Show me "The boy is playing."
>
> Client: (points to the correct picture)

With the task designed in this fashion, there is more evidence that the client understands the verb "play" or at least is able to differentiate it from the verb "cook." One would have to assess many different verbs and assess them in different combinations to be certain. Please remember our discussion in a previous section of this chapter that there is a high level of success from random selection when the field consists of only two choices.

Another way the original task can be altered is as follows:

> Clinician: (shows the client two pictures. In one, the boy is playing. In the other, the girl is cooking.) Show me "play."
>
> Client: (points to the correct picture)

Note that this presentation does not reflect much alteration of the original task. Thus, minor modification of the stimulus has resulted in an effective task. It does assess that which it was designed to do. Again, it is important to give adequate thought to tasks prior to presentation. In this manner, many sources of invalid responses can be anticipated and thus avoided.

QUICK CHECK

Make certain that your receptive tasks measure precisely what they were designed to measure. If the client correctly responds, it should be because he understands that which is being assessed.

PROBLEM AND SOLUTION 15: GROUPS

Beginning clinicians often work with groups of clients but do not perform group therapy. There is a definite distinction between "therapy in a group" and "group therapy." An example of "therapy in a group" is provided here. The goal of the session for the first client is to correctly produce the /s/ phoneme in the initial position of words. The second client's goal is to correctly produce the /s/ phoneme in the initial position of words in sentences. The example is:

Clinician: (showing the client a picture) What's this?

Client 1:   Sun.

Clinician: Good sound! This one? (shows picture)

Client 1:   Soap.

Clinician: Nice! Here's another. (shows picture)

Client 1:   Soup.

Clinician: Good job! It's Jimmy's turn now. (shows picture) Make a sentence.

Client 2:   The sink is dirty.

Clinician: Good! This one? (shows picture)

Client 2:   The sailboat is pretty.

Clinician: Super! One more. (shows picture)

Client 2:   The soda is cold.

Clinician: Nice work! It's Billy's [client 1's] turn.

It can easily be seen that this beginning clinician was providing individual therapy to each of the clients in a group setting. There was absolutely no interaction between the clients. Therefore, it might be more advantageous for each client to be seen for 15 minutes of individual therapy instead of one half hour of so-called group therapy. The clinician divided the time in half and was, in essence, devoting 15 minutes to each client. Thus, "therapy in a group," rather than "group therapy," was conducted.

Granted, actual "group therapy" is harder to plan and execute than individual therapy or "therapy in a group." There are two types of interaction that can occur during group therapy sessions. The first type of interaction is that which occurs on non–goal-related activities (one child selects pictures for the other child to say, one child monitors the other child's production, etc.). The second type of interaction occurs while working toward the therapy goals of the session. When clinicians are instructed to perform "group therapy," they incorporate interaction into their sessions. However, it is the first, and the easier, type that is implemented. An example is as follows:

Clinician: Johnny, here are Billy's cards. Billy, here are Johnny's card. Johnny, go first. Billy, show Johnny a card.

Billy: (shows a picture of a sun)

Johnny: <u>Sun</u>.

Clinician: Billy, was his sound good?

Billy: (nods head yes)

Clinician: Good work, boys! Johnny, show Billy a card.

Johnny: (shows a picture of a saddle)

Billy: <u>Saddle</u>.

Clinician: (looks at Johnny) Well?

Johnny: It was good.

Clinician: Nice job, boys!

Interaction was not observed on the actual goals of the session, but it did occur in other areas. Each client was actively involved throughout the entire session. When it was not the one client's turn to respond, he showed pictures to the other client and listened to his responses in order to state if they were correct or not. Another way in which clinicians frequently try to accomplish this first type of interaction is through the use of an activity board. They believe that interaction is obtained because the clients are moving various spaces on the same board. This type of interaction is better than none, but it leaves a lot to be desired in the actual implementation of group therapy.

The second type of interaction, although extremely desirable, is harder to achieve. Most beginning clinicians believe it cannot be obtained unless the clients are working on exactly the same goals. This is not necessarily so. The original example is redesigned to portray the idea of group therapy, as follows:

Clinician: (showing the client a picture) What's this?

Client 1:   Sun.

Clinician: Good sound! (looking at client 2) Make a sentence!

Client 2:   The sun is yellow.

Clinician: Good job! What's this? (looking at client 1)

Client 1:   Soap.

Clinician: Sounds good! How about a sentence? (looking at client 2)

Client 2:   I wash with soap.

Clinician: Nice!

Interaction was obtained on the goals of the session. The second client's responses build on those of the first client. This procedure could also be reversed. An example is:

Clinician: (showing the client a picture) Make a sentence!

Client 2:   The sun is yellow.

Clinician: Good! (looking at client 1) Which word has your sound?

Client 1:   Sun.

Clinician: How was it?

Client 1:   Good?

Clinician: Right!

It is possible to obtain both types of interaction in the same session. The example just given is now modified as follows:

Clinician: Billy, here are some pictures. Johnny, here are some pictures. Billy goes first. Johnny, show Billy a card.

Johnny: (shows a picture of a seal)

Billy: Seal.

Clinician: (looks at Johnny) Well?

Johnny: It was good.

Clinician: You're both right! Your turn. (looks at Johnny)

Johnny: The <u>seal</u> is black.

Billy: Sounded good! Show me another card. (looks at Johnny)

Strive to incorporate interaction, particularly the latter type, into your therapy sessions. Accept the challenge of providing "group therapy" rather than "therapy in a group."

QUICK CHECK

Analyze the dynamics of your group therapy. Are you really conducting "group therapy" or is it "therapy in a group?"

PROBLEM AND SOLUTION 16: HABITS THAT MAY BE MISINTERPRETED

Two of many habits discussed here can be interpreted as either signs of nervousness or boredom. When you are observed constantly swinging your leg under the table or twisting your hair, a feeling of nervousness is perceived. When you rest your head or chin on your hand, the idea of boredom is conveyed. It does not matter if you are or are not nervous or bored. These impressions should *not* be conveyed. Favorable impressions will not be received by clients, families of the clients on your caseload, or people observing you if these behaviors are present. In most cases, observation of your performance will continue throughout your professional career. Therefore, it is worth your effort to eliminate these negative behaviors now to help make a favorable, and professional, impression.

QUICK CHECK

Videotape a session if possible, after obtaining the necessary permission. Analyze the tape. Make certain you are not exhibiting signs of nervousness or boredom.

PROBLEM AND SOLUTION 17: THE GAME "MIRAGE"

If you do not want the client to respond "We played games" when his classroom teacher inquires, you must watch where the emphasis of the session is placed. Games and/or activities are frequently used to facilitate speech and language goals. They are a means to an end. You should place the emphasis on the speech- and language-related goals—not on the game or activity. You should not make comments such as the following: "Neither of you won because no one got to the end," "We don't have a winner again," "The first one to finish the game gets a prize," or "You both got to the witch's broom. Good job!" These comments definitely reflect a misplaced emphasis. If you do not want the client to say "We played games," the emphasis had better be quickly changed. Further, the client who "wins" the game should do so because he reached criterion on a particular objective and not solely because he rolled the higher numbers on the die. Let us view an excerpt from a therapy session. Correct production of the /r/ phoneme in the initial position of words was the goal. A portion of the session follows:

Clinician: Roll the die!

Client 1:   (rolls die) Five.

Clinician: What's this? (shows picture)

Client 1:   Rat.

Clinician: Good. Move five spaces. Your turn. (looking at client 2)

Client 2:   (rolls die) Three.

Clinician: (shows picture)

Client 2:   Radio.

Clinician: Nice! Move three spaces.

More emphasis can be placed on the actual goal of the session by making a slight modification. An example is:

Clinician: Roll the die!

Client 1:   (rolls die) Five.

Clinician: What are these? (shows pictures)

Client 1:   Rat, razor.

Clinician: Good! These?

Client 1: <u>R</u>ug, <u>rain</u>, <u>rabbit</u>.

Clinician: Good. You said five good /r/ sounds. Move five spaces. (passes die to client 2)

Client 2: Three.

Clinician: (shows pictures)

Client 2: <u>Rainbow</u>, <u>ribbon</u>. (distorted)

Clinician: Where's your good sound? Try that one again.

Client 2: <u>Ribbon</u>.

Clinician: That's better.

Client 2: <u>Robot</u>.

Clinician: You had two good /r/ sounds. Move two spaces.

Note that the client was made aware that moving spaces was contingent on correct production of the /r/ phoneme in words. In the first example, the client moved five spaces for saying one /r/ word correctly. In the second example, the client moved five spaces only if /r/ in five words was said correctly. A big difference between the first and second example is that the client was reminded of the goal (correct production of the /r/ phoneme in the initial position of words) throughout the activity in the latter example. There was no reference made to the goal in the first example. It is important to remember that the client's perception of the session, including the goal(s), is a reflection of the manner in which it is conducted.

QUICK CHECK

Make certain your emphasis of the session is appropriate. It should be placed on the goals of the session—not on games or activities.

PROBLEM AND SOLUTION 18: CARRYOVER

Professionals in the field of speech-language pathology frequently comment that obtaining carryover (generalization) is problematic. Carryover is the process of exhibiting newly learned techniques (correct production of a particular sound, use of present progressive tense, and so forth) in all situations regardless of the environment or the people present. Many clinicians complain that the client simply does not use the technique in question outside of the environment in which it was initially performed. This author has discovered that carryover or generalization is more likely to be attained when steps are taken to make the client more independent. It has been found that a client moves toward becoming independent if two aspects are emphasized as early as possible in the therapeutic program. *Monitoring* and *performing specific assignments* both lead to more client involvement and to more independence. In this way, the client becomes responsible for his own performance.

Monitoring

Monitoring should be encouraged to help the client move toward becoming independent. When a client begins working on a new goal, he should know the expectations. He should know when responses are correct and when they are not. Initially, you have to perform the monitoring function. If you continue to monitor, however, dependence can be perpetuated. Only when a client becomes aware that his behavior is or is not correct can change take place. If the client perceives his production as not being correct, he will try to correct it by making a change. If the client perceives his production as correct, he will try to stabilize it. Self-listening or monitoring should be emphasized as soon as therapy is started. Because there is a tendency to exclude monitoring, an example demonstrating this aspect is included.

Clinician: Johnny, say /s/.

Johnny: /θ/. (produces a frontal lisp)

Clinician: Close your teeth. Try again.

Johnny: (produces a distorted /s/)

Clinician: You're getting closer! Where should your tongue tip be?

Johnny: Here. (points)

Clinician: Yes. Try again /s/.

Johnny: /s/.

Clinician: Super! /s/

Johnny: /θ/. (produces a frontal lisp)

Clinician: How were your front teeth?

Johnny: Apart.

Clinician: How should they be?

Johnny: Together.

Clinician: Yes. Try again. /s/

Johnny: /s/.

Clinician: Did it sound right?

Johnny: Yes.

Clinician: Good. Say /s/.

Johnny: /θ/. (produces a frontal lisp)

Clinician: How was it?

Johnny: Not so hot.

Clinician: Why?

Johnny: My teeth weren't closed.

Clinician: Right you are!

It can be seen that the client is being prepared to monitor his productions and take responsibility for his therapeutic program right from the start. The client knows the characteristics of the target phoneme. When monitoring is first introduced, it may be somewhat time consuming. If the groundwork is done properly, monitoring will soon become automatic. An example is:

Clinician: Let's hear your sound.

Client: /s/. It sounded good.

Clinician: Right. Keep going.

Client: /s/; good. /s/; yes. /s/; good.

Clinician: Right you are!

Monitoring does not have to occur verbally. For example, two faces (a smiling face and a frowning face) can be placed in front of the client. The client points to the smiling face to indicate that his production was correct. He points to the frowning face to indicate that his production was not correct. Less time is consumed in this manner. Another example of a nonverbal monitoring system is to have a picture of a traffic light. The client points to "green" for a correct response and "red" for an incorrect response. Counters operating red and green lights can also be used. The client can press the lever on the counter with the green light for a correct response and the lever with the red light for an incorrect response. A client can monitor responses in numerous ways. The important aspect is that the system used be appropriate for the client's level.

Whatever type of monitoring system is established, one must be certain that the client is *actively* listening and evaluating each production rather that simply saying "good" or pointing to the smiling face in an automatic fashion. The extra time taken to establish a monitoring system in the very early sessions of the therapy program is definitely worthwhile because the client will become more independent, and, as a result, progress will be more rapid.

Assignments

To ensure carryover, assignments should be implemented as soon as appropriate. It is not necessary to wait for mastery before instructing the client to practice the new behavior in other environments and with other people. For example, if a client is working on correct production of the /s/ phoneme in isolation, you do not have to wait until /s/ is correctly produced in conversation before attempting to obtain carryover. Various substeps, as small and/or insignificant as they seem, can be made into worthwhile assignments. For example, if the client is having difficulty producing /s/ in isolation, practicing production would not be realistic or helpful at this point. The client could, however, be given an assignment leading up to the accomplishment of the objective, as long as it was related to the objective, was preliminary in nature, and the client had the necessary capabilities. In the case of a client who substitutes θ/s, focusing on keeping his front teeth together is a definite step toward accomplishment of the objective. Therefore, a possible substep is to have the client look in a mirror and make certain that his front teeth are together. This can be made into an assignment.

This author has found that assignments are more likely to be completed or at least attempted by the client if two conditions exist. First, the assignment must be specific. Second, there must be a way to check the client's performance. An example of a specific assignment is "Everyday until our next session, look in the mirror three times a day—around breakfast, dinner, and bedtime. Put your front teeth together lightly but without tension five times." The first condition, a specific assignment, was met. What about the second condition, a way to check the client's performance? This can be met by designing a check sheet. An example is:

Assignment
(front teeth together lightly without tension)

	Tuesday	Wednesday
Breakfast	1 2 3 4 5	1 2 3 4 5
Dinner	1 2 3 4 5	1 2 3 4 5
Bedtime	1 2 3 4 5	1 2 3 4 5

Key: X = correct; O = incorrect.

Done in this manner, it is possible to determine how the client performed by glancing at the completed check sheet. A client is much more likely to perform an assignment of this nature for many reasons. He has a check sheet, an actual piece of paper, that serves as a reminder. In addition, the client has to put an "X" on the number of the attempt if it was performed correctly or an "O" if performed incorrectly. The client also has to return the assignment to the clinician the next session. For these reasons, the client will more than likely attempt, and complete, the assignment.

On the other hand, because the client was given an assignment, it is your responsibility to review it at the beginning of the next session. If the client does not automatically give you the check sheet, ask for it. Quickly scan and calculate the client's performance. Ask if the client had any difficulty. Reinforce the client in an age-appropriate manner for completion of the assignment.

Problems that beginning clinicians have with assignments are numerous. One of the most common is that assignments are not specific. An example of a nonspecific assignment for a client starting to correctly produce /s/ in conversation is:

Clinician: Remember to work on /s/.

It is obvious that this is vague. What exactly is the client to do? How often should the client do it? With whom should it be done? In what environment? Another problem is that this beginning clinician had no way to determine whether the client had success.

Yet another problem deals with the lack of follow-through on the clinician's part. This occurs when the clinician gives an assignment but does not take the time to see whether the client completed it or to determine how the client performed. Because of this lack of follow-through, the client may get the idea that assignments are not important and conclude that there is no reason to do them.

It is important to remember and implement other information into your assignments that will help promote carryover. Use situations and materials from the client's life, as these will be more functional and will have a greater impact. Be certain to vary the setting as well as the listeners and speakers as appropriate.

QUICK CHECK

Have immediate success with carryover! Make certain you implement monitoring and the use of specific assignments as early as appropriate in the therapeutic process.

PROBLEM AND SOLUTION 19: DOING TOO MUCH WORK

I know this problem has certainly caught your attention. You have been thinking this ever since your clinical practicum days started. There are ways that *some* of your work can be eliminated. One day, I went into our "clinic room" where our student clinicians gather. One student was frantically looking through a dictionary and making a list of words. I asked what she was doing. She said she was preparing for her next therapy session. She was working with a university student who had a frontal lisp. There was no reason why this beginning clinician had to construct a word list. Some of this responsibility should have been placed on the client. One way in which this can be done is through an assignment. For example:

Clinician: Your next session is Thursday. Make a list of 25 new words beginning with /s/. Bring it with you. You'll practice them next time.

Additionally, if you are working with a 5-year-old client on the production of /p/ in the initial position of words, you do not have to think of all the stimulus words. Remember, you want the client to be responsible for his therapy and you want the family to get involved. Therefore, you can put some of the responsibility of thinking of stimulus words on the client and his family. For example, you can give an assignment of this nature.

Clinician: (hands the client a paper bag from the supermarket) Look around your house. Find 12 objects that begin with your /p/ sound. Put them in this bag and bring it next time.

In this manner, some of the responsibility for stimulus materials for the next session has been shifted to the client and his family.

> ## QUICK CHECK
>
> Make your clients responsible for their stimulus words and materials when appropriate!

PROBLEM AND SOLUTION 20: SIGN LANGUAGE

Beginning clinicians frequently approach the teaching of signs as a totally new and unique experience. Other than possibly learning new signs, this should not be a source of concern for you. You are familiar with language theory and language therapy, and it is this information that forms the basis for "teaching" sign language. Before an explanation is given, a portion of a therapy session is explored. Single quotation marks indicate that the contents were signed.

Clinician: (shows a picture) What is the dog doing?

Client: (makes inappropriate sign)

Clinician: No, here's 'sleep.' You try.

Client: 'Sleep.' (imitates sign correctly)

Clinician: That's right! What is the girl doing?

Client: 'Swim.'

Clinician: Good! What is the man doing?

Client: 'Eat.'

Clinician: Good job!

A few changes are necessary to make this session and the clinician's approach productive and effective. First, it is important to remember that language is divided into receptive and expressive modalities. The receptive modality is frequently overlooked when teaching sign language. It must be remembered that if a client is going to use sign language to communicate (the ultimate goal), he must also be able to understand or "read" the signs of others when they communicate. Also if you recall learning signs, it was more difficult to "read" the signs of others than to use them for communication. Therefore, the client should be exposed to the receptive modality first. Pictures depicting the various actions in the sample just given should be placed in front of the client. The clinician should sign one of the verbs. This should be followed by the client's receptive identification of the appropriate picture.

Another change is that this clinician should simultaneously sign everything said to the client. One must remember that it is through signs that this client will communicate. Expanding and modeling should be done in the same manner as with "normal" clients and those with specific language impairments. Expanding and modeling must always be appropriate to the level at which the client is functioning. These changes are reflected in the following excerpt:

Clinician: (places three pictures in front of the client) Swim. Point to swim.

Client: (points to the correct picture)

Clinician: Good! Girl swim. (removes and replaces picture) Sleep. Where's sleep?

Client: (points to the correct picture)

Clinician: Yes. Dog sleep.

QUICK CHECK

Treat sign language as you do language. Remember, there is also a receptive modality. It is important for the client to be able to "read" signs.

PROBLEM AND SOLUTION 21: SESSION OPENING

Beginning clinicians tend to forget to "open" their sessions. Sessions should begin with someone stating the goal(s). That someone will be either you or the client, depending on the circumstances. If the client has been involved with the therapeutic process for a while and if the client is capable, the client should take an active role in the opening. He can state what he is working on. Examples are:

Clinician: What are you working on?

Client: Is verbing.

———

Clinician: What is your sound?

Client: /s/.

If the client is just beginning the therapeutic process or if the goal(s) of the session is changing, then it will be necessary for you to specifically state the goal(s) of the session. This should be done in terminology the client can understand. Ideally, the stating of the session's goal(s) is the client's responsibility.

QUICK CHECK

Ask yourself, "Do I have a session opening? Am I encouraging the client to take an active role in it?"

PROBLEM AND SOLUTION 22: SESSION CLOSING

Warning

Part of closing a session includes providing the client with notice that the session is almost over. It is necessary to address this aspect, as beginning clinicians have a tendency to end their therapy sessions abruptly. An example is:

Clinician: Make a sentence.

Client: The dog ran after the cat.

Clinician: Time is up. See you next week. (hands client his notebook; stands up)

This ending needs to be improved for many reasons. Many clinicians have tried very hard to get clients to enjoy therapy and have been successful in doing so. Many clients do like therapy, look forward to their sessions, and do not like to see them end. Therefore, if "warnings" that the session is going to end are given in advance, it makes the ending easier for the client to accept. Several examples of warnings are given below:

Clinician: Five more sentences. Then it will be time to go.

———

Clinician: Make a sentence for each of these pictures (shows the client the amount of pictures). Then we're done.

———

Clinician: Two more minutes and then it's time to go.

The actual "warning" given must be appropriate to the client's level of functioning. For example, if the client does not understand numbers, telling him "five more sentences" would not be appropriate. If the client does not understand the concept of time, then saying "two more minutes" would not be appropriate. Showing the client how many more he has to complete would be appropriate if he does not understand the concept of time or numbers. These are only a few suggestions. The possibilities of informing the client that the session is ending are numerous.

Wrap-up

It is important that the session end on a positive note so that the client feels good about himself as well as his accomplishment. If the client did not have much success during the session, it may be necessary to end with an easier task—one on which you know the client can succeed. In this manner, the client will have something positive to feel good about.

It is also important that the client has a good understanding of his therapeutic program. To make certain the client knows the goal(s) of the session, it (they) should be reviewed at the end of the session. Ideally, this review should be done by the client. If this is not possible (for reasons already provided in the section "Session Opening"), then you should provide the review.

Clinician Example

Clinician: Today you worked on /s/ at the end of words.

Client Example

Clinician: What did you work on today?

Client: My /s/ sound.

QUICK CHECK

Make certain you have adequate session closure. Provide a specific warning that the session is about to end. The goals should be reviewed. Be certain the client takes an active role in this review when applicable.

CONCLUSION

In this chapter, many suggestions to improve or enhance performance during the therapeutic process were provided. Modification of seating arrangements that decreased distractions and assisted with record-keeping functions were discussed. The importance of effective usage of reinforcement was emphasized. Differences in reinforcement techniques were noted for use in therapy and evaluations. Implications of accidental and/or inappropriate reinforcement were given, and examples were provided. Clinicians were encouraged to present good verbal models. Usage of the "OK syndrome," unnatural production of words, ungrammatical utterances, and utterances that foster dependency should be eliminated. Language should be modeled at a level commensurate with or slightly above, but not far beyond, the client's current linguistic functioning.

When presenting choices, the number must be kept constant. In this manner, the probability of correct responses occurring by chance remains equal. When choices involve pictures or objects, they should be presented to the client in natural reading sequence, which, in English, is left to right, top to bottom.

All tasks should receive serious thought and consideration before being presented. Will the expressive task really elicit the desired or target structure? If not, redesign the task. Always be certain that the expected response is both normal and appropriate to the situation. Make certain that receptive tasks really measure that which they were designed to measure.

When working with groups, accept the challenge of providing "group therapy" and not just "therapy in a group." Other suggestions to keep in mind are to eliminate habits that may be perceived as portraying nervousness or boredom. Place the emphasis of the session where it belongs—on the speech, language, and communication aspects and not on games or activities. To assist the client with accepting responsibility for his problem and his therapy program, begin to implement monitoring behavior during the initial stages of his therapy program. It is only when a client is aware of the incorrectness of a response that change can be made.

It is hoped that some of the information contained in this chapter was mentally applied to either sessions you have observed or sessions you have conducted. It is also hoped that this information will be applied to future sessions. If you are receptive and eager to learn as much as possible, this chapter has provided a head start. Duplication of the errors of your predecessors should not occur, as you can learn from them. Awareness of the pitfalls has been heightened. Examples, explanations, and solutions have been provided. Take advantage of this opportunity, and strive to develop to your fullest potential!

KNOW IT! USE IT!

After reading this chapter, you should be able to:

1. demonstrate an optimal seating arrangement while conducting therapy as determined by your supervisor
2. demonstrate appropriate usage of reinforcement techniques in 90% of the obligatory contexts as determined by your supervisor
3. state three problems that frequently occur with verbal models
4. demonstrate correct modeling behavior in 90% of the obligatory contexts as determined by your supervisor
5. state and explain without error eight cues and/or prompts used to elicit correct production of errored phonemes starting with those providing the maximum amount of support
6. give a correct example of "group therapy" as determined by your supervisor
7. demonstrate techniques to get the client to monitor his responses in 90% of the obligatory contexts
8. state two ways to ensure carry-over
9. present clear, precise, concise directions in 90% of your attempts as determined by your supervisor

REFERENCES

Bain, B. (1994). A framework for dynamic assessment in phonology: Stimulability revisited. *Clinics in Communication Disorders, 4*(1), 12–22.

Leahy, M. (1995). *Disorders of communication: The science of intervention.* London: Whurr Publishers.

McDonald, E.T. (1964). *A deep test of articulation.* Pittsburgh, PA: Stanwix House.

Miller, J.F. (1981). *Assessing language production in children.* Baltimore, MD: University Park Press.

Reed, V. (1994). *An introduction to children with language disorders* (2nd ed.). New York: Macmillan.

Chapter 8

Self-Evaluation: "Mirror, Mirror"

CHAPTER HIGHLIGHTS

- *the importance of self-evaluation*
- *techniques used to assist with self-evaluation*
- *basic clinical behaviors to include in a self-evaluation*
- *complex clinical behaviors to include in a self-evaluation*

Anderson (1988b) brilliantly conveys the tone for the importance of self-evaluation:

> Supervision must be more than just waiting for someone else to decide what is right and what is wrong. It requires the highest levels of insight about oneself and the other participants. It means action based on that insight. It requires study of the process and, most of all, . . . study of self. (p. viii)

It is important for you to evaluate continually all aspects of your professional performance. This self-evaluation, or, as it is sometimes called, self-assessment, self-supervision, or self-observation, should begin as early as possible during the clinical experience and, according to Anderson (1988a), is the most advanced stage of supervision. At the beginning, however, you will rely on your supervisor to provide most of the feedback as well as a great deal of direction. This practice was formalized by Van Riper (1965) in his prescription that "initial sessions with beginning clinicians should be highly structured by the supervisor" but that "supervisory input should fade as the clinician gains in experience" (p. 324). How much supervision is required at the beginning and how quickly independence is acquired are determined by hours of experience, number of clients served, experience with the disorder area, experience with the therapeutic approach, practicum site, the clinician's academic performance, and the clinician's progress in clinical performance.

The position statement of the American Speech-Language-Hearing Association (ASHA, 1985) on the role of clinical supervision in speech-language pathology and audiology reads:

> A central premise of supervision is that effective clinical teaching involves, in a fundamental way, the development of self-analysis, self-evaluation, and problem-solving skills on the part of the individual being supervised. The success of clinical teaching rests largely on the achievement of this goal. (p. 57)

Casey, Smith, & Ulrich (1988, p. 27) state:

> Self-supervision is a life-long professional goal and not something that ends with a semester or when a particular supervisory interaction concludes. It is a behavior that will continue and evolve across supervisors, work settings, and clients throughout professional careers. There are many purposes for engaging in self-supervision. The most important include:

1. to assess strengths and needs
2. to facilitate development of clinical and supervisory skills
3. to understand clinical interactions (i.e., clinician effect on client behavior and client effect on clinician behavior)
4. to understand intraprofessional (within the profession) interactions (i.e., clinician effects on supervisor and or colleagues, supervisor effect on clinician or others)
5. to understand interprofessional (outside the profession) interactions (e.g., non–speech-language pathology or audiology supervisor or administrator, or other health care or education professionals)
6. to assure accountability in both the clinical and supervisory processes
7. to understand issues and be aware of resources related to self-supervision

Being able to evaluate or analyze your own performance accurately and realistically and make indicated changes is a giant step toward achieving independent clinical functioning because services are often provided without supervision. Early development of the necessary skills to take on the role of being your own supervisor is, therefore, very important. Equally important is the commitment to improve and upgrade your skills continuously for the duration of your professional career. Casey, Smith, and Ulrich (1988) stated, "Each [speech-language pathologist] continues to engage in some form of supervision as a career-long activity" (p. xii). Therefore, it is extremely important to develop good self-evaluation skills early in your career.

INITIAL SELF-EVALUATIONS

It has been observed that "beginning clinicians are more often concerned about what 'to do' next time and not [with] the how or why procedures" (Brasseur and Jimenez, 1994, p. 113). If this remains your focus, you will not develop good self-evaluation skills. Your evaluation will be shallow. It is necessary to learn to analyze all aspects of the session as well as your performance critically and in-depth.

There is a strong probability that your initial evaluations of your clinical performance will be shallow and uninteresting. In response to a request for clinicians to assess a therapy session, frequently elicited comments are "It was a good session," "I feel good about the session," "It was an OK session," "It could have been better," or "It wasn't very good." It is obvious that these "evaluations" lack substance. Rationales are not provided to explain why the session was "good," "OK," or "not very good."

When examined further, these session evaluations appear to be based on whether the client was interested in the task or materials, or whether the client changed his speech and/or language behavior. These "evaluations" do not often contain information about your behaviors. Self-reporting or disclosure may, ironically, be most valuable when a client does not make progress or when a session does not go well. In these cases, you need to examine your own behavior thoroughly before placing blame elsewhere. You may sometimes act in a manner that blocks expected progress or prevents the session from being "good." Careful evaluations can determine what went wrong and what changes need to be implemented to improve the next session. To do this, good self-evaluation skills are essential.

SELF-OBSERVATION TECHNIQUES

To evaluate behavior, it is first necessary to observe behavior. Bernthal and Beukelman (1975, p. 40) define observation as the "recording of clinical behaviors." They go on to say that there are three observation techniques that can be used for evaluating performance: audio recording, video recording, or recording by an observer. If it is at all possible, you should use audio or video devices (after appropriate consent is obtained) as early as practical in the progression toward becoming your own supervisor. These tapes should be reviewed with chapter 7 in mind and in light of any existing supervisory comments. Dowling (1992) agrees that videotaping is valuable. Observing videotapes of your sessions enables you to step outside yourself and learn not only about yourself but also the impact you have on the client's performance. You will be able to determine aspects of the session that went well and identify aspects that need to be improved. You may be able to develop your evaluation skills further if, occasionally, you invite your supervisor or a peer to observe a portion of the videotape in order to obtain a different viewpoint.

Introspective self-observation can be instituted at this time or, most certainly, later. This undertaking—looking at oneself with objective detachment—is not easy for most people; however, it can help tremendously. Starting with a review of the indices discussed next, one can discern trends across clients having similar presenting problems. Later, you can fine tune this analysis by using the instruments appearing later in this chapter.

INITIAL FOCUS: BENCHMARK MEASUREMENTS

You will be better able to evaluate your therapy sessions and your own performance when provided with specific direction. Bernthal and Beukelman (1975) give six aspects of clinical behavior that can be used to evaluate a session. Each is stated, summarized, and discussed here.

1. Determining Participation Percentages and Patterns

Because a therapy session is limited in time, every minute must focus on remediation of the client's problem. Time must be used efficiently and effectively. It is not in the client's best interest for the session to be dominated by irrelevant interchanges, socializing, or other behaviors that are not geared toward direct remediation. Extraneous interchange limits available time for the client to work on the therapeutic objectives and to make necessary changes.

Participation percentages may be calculated in one of two ways. The focus is placed on *the number of words* spoken by you and the client or on the *amount of time* spoken by you and the client. If the number of words spoken is the focus, they are counted during a segment of therapy that is representative of the session. (Here, an audio recording is a big help.) The participation percentage is calculated by dividing the number of words spoken by each person by the total number of words produced during the segment and multiplying by 100. The formula is:

$$\frac{\text{Number of Words Spoken by Client}}{\text{Total Number of Words Produced}} \times 100 = \text{Participation Percentage}$$

If the focus is placed on the amount of time spoken by you and the client, it is best to audiotape the session. Select a representative segment of the session. Play the tape and determine the amount of time you talk, as well as the amount of time the client talks. Determine the total time of the segment. The participation percentage is calculated by dividing the amount of time spoken by each person by the segment's total amount of time and multiplying by 100. The formula is:

$$\frac{\text{Amount of Time Client Talks}}{\text{Total Amount of All Talking Time}} \times 100 = \text{Participation Percentage}$$

This information, calculated for words or time, will show if you are monopolizing the session. It must be remembered that if the client is not participating, speech and/ or language behavior is not changing.

2. Determining Response Rate of Target Behaviors

This information will enable you to determine whether a particular therapeutic technique results in obtaining a desired number of responses per minute. "Mowrer (1973) recommends that response rates should average between 15 and 25 responses per minute during the initial phases of articulation instruction and between 6 and 10 responses per minute during connected speech or carry-over activities" (cited in Bernthal & Beukelman, 1975, p. 41). Usually, a professional half-hour therapy session is actually 25 minutes in length. Therefore, based on Mowrer's numbers given above, between 375 and 625 responses per session should be obtained during the initial phases of articulation instruction and between 150 and 250 responses per session should be obtained during connected speech or carry-over activities (assuming the entire session is devoted to these tasks). The response rate is determined by dividing the number of client responses produced by the number of minutes in the session. If, however, different tasks are performed in a session, individual response rates should be obtained for each. It is best to calculate an overall response rate as well as individual response rates for each task.

In a later study, Mowrer (1988) identified both clinician and client behaviors associated with low- and high-target response rates. Clinicians' behaviors associated with low response rates were "talking about subjects which were unrelated to evoking the target response (social interchanges, homework assignments, game instructions, etc.), re-instructing children who failed to repeat all the words of [the] sentence model, and ignoring children who were silent" (p. 107). Children's behaviors associated with low response rates were:

> talking about subjects unrelated to the target response (social interchange), watching others perform motor tasks such as those performed in game and playing activities, listening to various auditory stimuli (others responding, word discrimination), and performing motor tasks which were unrelated to producing the target response (drawing cards, opening easter eggs, cutting and pasting, etc.). (p. 107)

On the other hand, clinicians' behaviors related to high response rates were "presenting picture cues containing the target sound, [and] presenting auditory cues containing the target sound" (p. 107). The only children's behavior identified that was associated with a high response rate was "replying to the teacher's instructions to name or repeat a word or phrase containing the target sound" (p. 107).

3. Determining Percentage of Correct Responses

One way of measuring a client's success on a task is to determine the percentage of correct responses. This is done by dividing the number of correct responses by the total number of responses (correct and incorrect) on a designated task and multiplying by 100. Mowrer (1988) analyzed behaviors of clinicians associated with low- and high-accuracy rates. Only one clinician behavior relating to a high accuracy rate was cited: "recognition of a correct response when that response was correct" (p. 108). Clinician behaviors related to a low accuracy rate were "A. Providing verbal praise ('Good') following an incorrect response. B. Presenting tasks beyond the child's skill level. C. Ignoring a correct response." (p. 108)

4. Determining Accuracy of Reinforcement

Reinforcement is an extremely powerful tool in modifying speech and/or language behavior. It is extremely important to reinforce promptly and accurately. A continuous reinforcement schedule is one in which all correct responses are reinforced. This type of schedule is most effective for establishing new behaviors. Once a behavior is established, a change in reinforcement is necessary. You should change from a continuous schedule to a type of intermittent schedule that is best to maintain behaviors. Intermittent reinforcement schedules provide "greater resistance to extinction" (Mowrer, 1988, p. 209).

You should evaluate your behavior to determine two things. The first deals with the number of accurate reinforcement sequences. That is, is the target behavior promptly followed by a reinforcer? The second deals with the inaccurate reinforcement sequence. That is, is the target behavior followed by no reinforcement or is the reinforcer given when no correct response occurs? Because of the importance of reinforcement, all clinicians should strive for perfection in this area.

5. Comparing the Instructional Plan to the Behavioral Record

Before the initiation of the session, a lesson plan (instructional plan) is developed (see chapter 2). After the session, what was done in the session (behavioral record) should be reviewed to determine whether the instructional plan was followed or if activities other than those specified were implemented. If deviation from the plan occurred, the clinician must be able to justify all changes. If a clinician finds that there is frequent deviation from the plan, the method of developing the plan should be examined. Flexibility is desirable, but it must be explained.

6. Systematic Recording of Client Behavior

Because it is necessary for you to know if the client's behavior is changing, it is important to keep accurate records on the client's behavior. Records on the number of correct and incorrect responses on each target behavior must be carefully and regularly kept and reviewed. Bernthal and Beukelman (1975) say these records make it possible to "determine the time frame in which the client changes his behavior, determine the behavioral change patterns associated with specific instructional procedures, and determine the learning curves associated with several procedures designed to teach the same target behavior" (p. 43).

In sum, to perform a self-evaluation adequately, it is necessary to calculate and review the indices just described. These six suggestions, however, are not ends in themselves but are an attempt to present you with concrete ways to start evaluating your performance. It is hoped that you can make use of these suggestions to avoid shallow and nondirective self-reviews. This is just the beginning of the path to developing accurate self-evaluation skills—a path that should never end.

LATER FOCUS: FINE TUNING CLINICAL COMPETENCE

When you can accurately evaluate your performance using Bernthal and Beukelman's (1975) six aspects of performance and make positive changes when warranted, it is time to focus on evaluating other more complex clinical behaviors that are expected by supervisors. Because these behaviors are more abstract, they will not be as easy to evaluate as those included in the initial focus.

The **Wisconsin Procedure for Appraisal of Clinical Competence (W-PACC)**, designed by Shriberg et al. (1975), is a very comprehensive instrument created to appraise "the extent to which effectiveness is dependent upon continued supervisory input" (p. 160). This instrument focuses on three categories: interpersonal skills, professional-technical skills, and personal qualities. Although different terms may be used by others to describe these three categories, these are the behaviors that supervisors deem important to develop and later evaluate in beginning clinicians. All categories are equally important, but there are more behaviors addressed under the professional-technical skills domain. This is because four major subdomains (developing and planning, teaching, assessment, and reporting) are included in this domain.

The **Clinician Appraisal Form,** a part of the **W-PACC**, is quite comprehensive in terms of the behaviors on which beginning clinicians should be evaluated. Because these are the behaviors that clinical supervisors assess, these are the behaviors that you should be using to evaluate yourself in order to improve your performance. There are 10 items on the "interpersonal skills" scale. According to Anderson (1988a), these items "appraise the clinician's ability to relate to and interact with the client, the client's family, and other professionals in a manner which is conducive to effective management" (p. 340). These items (pp. 349–350) are:

1. accepts, empathizes, shows genuine concern for the client as a person and understands the client's problems, needs, and stresses
2. perceives verbal and nonverbal cues which indicate the client is not understanding the task, is unable to perform all or part of the task, or is experiencing emotional stress that interferes with performance of the task
3. creates an atmosphere based on honesty and trust; enables client to express his/her feelings and concerns
4. conveys to the client in a nonthreatening manner what the standards of behavior and performance are
5. develops understanding of teaching goals and procedures with clients
6. listens, asks questions, participates *with* supervisor in therapy and/or client related discussions; is not defensive
7. requests assistance from supervisor and/or other professionals when appropriate
8. creates an atmosphere based on honesty and trust, enabling family members to express their feelings and concerns

9. develops understanding of teaching goals and procedures with family members

10. communicates with other disciplines on a professional level

The "professional-technical skills" scale comprises 28 items. The subdomain, "developing and planning," is composed of eight items. These items deal with your approach to the task. They are, according to Anderson (1988a, pp. 351–352):

1. applies academic information to the clinical process
2. researches problems and obtains pertinent information from supplemental reading and/or observing other clients with similar problems
3. develops a semester management program (conceptualized or written) appropriate to the client's needs
4. on the basis of assessment and measurement can appropriately determine measurable teaching objectives
5. plans appropriate teaching procedures
6. selects appropriate stimulus materials (age and ability level of client)
7. sequences teaching tasks to implement designated program objectives
8. plans strategies for maintaining on-task behavior (including structuring the teaching environment and setting behavioral limits)

The subdomain, "teaching," consists of nine items. These items are geared toward your ability to modify behavior. The items, according to Anderson (1988a, pp. 353–354), are:

9. gives clear, concise instructions in presenting materials and/or techniques in management and assessments
10. modifies level of language according to the needs of the client
11. utilizes planned teaching procedures
12. is adaptable—makes modifications in the teaching strategy such as shifting materials and/or techniques when the client is not understanding or performing the task
13. uses feedback and/or reinforcement that is consistent, discriminating, and meaningful to the client
14. selects pertinent information to convey to the client
15. maintains on-task behavior
16. prepares clinical setting to meet individual client and observer needs
17. if mistakes are made in the therapy situation, is able to generate ideas of what might have improved the situation

The next subdomain, "assessment," comprises seven items that focus on your ability to assess behavior and make recommendations. According to Anderson (1988a, pp. 354–355), these items are:

18. continues to assess client throughout the course of therapy using observational recording and standardized and nonstandardized measurement procedures and techniques
19. administers diagnostic tests according to standardization criterion
20. prepares prior to administering diagnostic tests by (a) having appropriate materials available [or] (b) gaining familiarity with testing procedures
21. scores diagnostic tests accurately
22. interprets results of diagnostic testing accurately
23. interprets accurately results of diagnostic testing in light of other available information to form an impression
24. makes appropriate recommendations and/or referrals based on information obtained from the assessment or teaching process

"Reporting" is the next subdomain. It consists of four items dealing with ability to formulate oral and written reports. According to Anderson (1988a, pp. 355–356), these items are:

25. reports information in written form that is pertinent and accurate
26. writes in an organized, concise, clear, and grammatically correct style
27. selects pertinent information to convey to family members
28. selects pertinent information to convey to other professionals (including all nonwritten communication such as phone calls and conferences)

The last 10 items pertain to the "personal qualities" domain and "provide additional information about the clinicians' general responsibility in clinical tasks" (p. 340). According to Anderson (1988a, p. 357), they are:

1. is punctual for client appointments
2. cancels client appointments when necessary
3. keeps appointments with supervisor or cancels appointments when necessary
4. turns in lesson plans on time
5. meets deadlines for reports
6. turns in attendance sheets on time
7. respects confidentiality of all professional activities
8. uses socially acceptable voice, speech, and language

9. presents appropriate personal appearance for clinical setting and maintaining credibility

10. appears to recognize own professional limitations and stays within boundaries of training

Clinicians receive numerical ratings, when applicable, on each item on the "interpersonal skills" and "professional-technical skills" scales. A rating of "1" is interpreted as "Specific direction from supervisor does not alter unsatisfactory performance and inability to make changes" (Anderson, 1988a, p. 356). The description, "Needs specific direction and/or demonstration from supervisor to perform effectively" (Anderson, 1988a, p. 356) is rated "2", "3," or "4" depending on performance. A rating of "5," "6," or "7" is earned if a clinician "needs general direction from supervisor to perform effectively" (Anderson, 1988a, p. 356) whereas an "8," "9," or "10" is earned if the clinician "demonstrates independence by taking initiative; makes changes when appropriate; and is effective" (Anderson, 1988a, p. 356). Items in the "personal qualities" domain are not numerically rated but are scaled in five categories: "does not apply," "lack information," "unsatisfactory," "inconsistent," and "satisfactory" (Anderson, 1988a, p. 357). If any of these items need clarification, descriptors are provided for all interpersonal items and professional-technical items in the original source or in Anderson (1988a).

ADDITIONAL STRATEGIES TO FACILITATE SELF-EVALUATION

Susann Dowling (1992) addresses additional strategies that you can use, independent of your supervisor, to gain control over your growth in the area of self-evaluation.

Familiarity with the Clinical Evaluation Form

One strategy involves becoming thoroughly familiar with the behaviors listed on the clinical evaluation form used at your university. Use this form as a checklist to plan your therapy session. Make certain that you address all the necessary areas. After your therapy session, complete the clinical evaluation form with regard to your behavior. This will help you "focus on the specific subcomponents of therapy and stimulates thought in regard to the clinical process" (Dowling, 1992, p. 254). On the basis of your evaluation, you will either continue your therapy in the same manner or make modifications for the next session. If your supervisor has observed and evaluated your session by completing the clinical evaluation form, you can further develop your evaluation skills by comparing the results before receiving additional supervisory feedback. This comparison provides valuable insight into the accuracy of your perceptions. As you become better able to analyze your performance accurately, more agreement will be found between your results and your supervisor's.

Observation of More Experienced Clinicians

To further your own clinical growth, it is advantageous to observe therapy sessions conducted by clinicians with more experience than you or who excel in an area in which you are having difficulty, as it will serve to increase the depth and extent of your experience. Dowling (1992) suggests that you "may also learn clinical flexibility, in discovering that a variety of options exist for achieving a specific goal." (pp. 254–255) These observations will also help you "build an internal concept of what constitutes successful therapy" (Dowling, 1992, p. 255) and will help build a knowledge base on which to evaluate your own performance.

Utilization of Peers

Peers can be instrumental in helping you develop your evaluation skills. Various issues can be discussed with colleagues. You may be able to extract some of this information and apply it to your functioning in the clinical setting. You can also observe a therapy session or a videotape of a peer's session. Together you can identify strengths as well as areas that need to be developed. Strategies for future sessions can be brainstormed. Getting insight from another person can only serve to increase your knowledge base and consequently give you additional ways to evaluate your own clinical performance (Dowling, 1992).

STUDENT SELF-APPRAISAL

"Student Self-Appraisal is a formalised procedure which enables students to self-evaluate and reflect on their clinical experience," according to McLeod (1994, p. 98). It encourages you to evaluate your performance and identify your strengths as well as the areas that need to be changed. "It provides a forum for students to take control of their own learning and to develop their own learning goals" (McLeod, 1994, p. 99). The Student Self-Appraisal focuses on a structured discussion between you and your supervisor. These discussions deal with your clinical placement and experience in a broad sense and do not predominantly focus on performance during the most recent clinical interaction as most meetings with supervisors do. As a result of these discussions, make a list of goals you want to achieve as well as a list of accomplishments that you have already achieved. A series of questions and probes are used to assist you with reflecting on your clinical placement. The first two questions deal with the positive aspects of your clinical experience: 1. "What have been the most satisfying aspects of your placement over this review period? What have been the high points?" (p. 101) and 2. "What do you consider are the most important activities you have performed over this review period?" (p.101). You then comment on your present caseload in question 3, which is "What do you think of the quantity and variety of your caseload?" (p. 101). Question 4, "What are the activities you would like to be doing that you are presently unable to do? What other tasks or roles would you like to try?" (p. 101) leads you to address other responsibilities you would like to undertake. Negative aspects of the clinical experience are addressed in the next question: "What are the particular difficulties/frustrations you have encountered in this placement? What have you done to improve them? What else can be done?" (p. 101). In question 6, you comment on the supervision received, when asked, "What further ways could you see your clinical educator facilitating your clinical work and satisfaction" (p. 101). Opportunities for self-development are the focus of question 7, when you are asked to "comment on the opportunities provided for your ongoing education and self-development" (p. 101). The last question provides you with the opportunity to discuss any other aspects about which you have concerns.

These discussions run for a minimum of 30 minutes and a maximum of 1 hour. You are to think about the questions and answer them in writing prior to your scheduled appointment. Your written responses are not given to your supervisor but serve as a way of getting yourself prepared and organized for the meeting. These Student Self-Appraisal meetings are conducted twice during each clinical experience—once at the midpoint and again at the end. The outcome of these Student Self-Appraisals are not supposed to be linked to a grade.

In a follow-up survey to determine the effectiveness of this procedure, positive comments were evident. Students said, "Student Self-Appraisal enables an objective examination of my skills"; "Student Self-Appraisal forces me to reflect on my clinical experiences"; " and "Student Self-Appraisal encourages problem solving" (McLeod, 1994, p. 94). Given the positive impact this procedure made on the students involved, it would be in your best interest to continue to reflect on your experience in this manner (Figure 8–1).

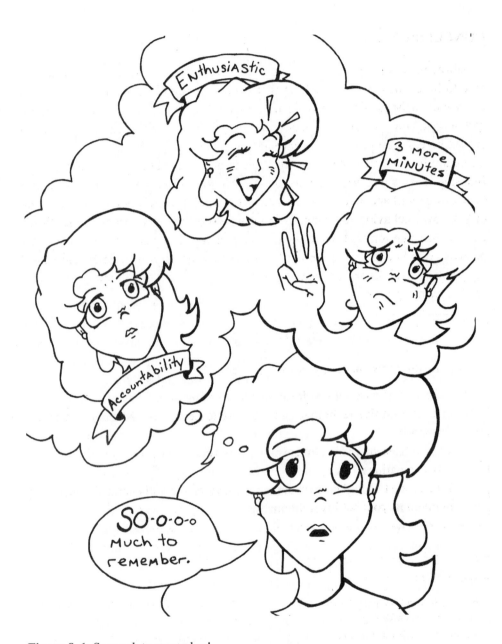

Figure 8–1 So much to remember!

CONCLUSION

Self-evaluation is an extremely important part of the clinical process. It is necessary to be cognizant of everything that occurs during client interactions. If you know what behaviors and/or skills are important in the role of a speech-language pathologist, you can strive to become competent in those areas. The behaviors discussed here are those deemed important by supervisors and, therefore, are those important for you to master. Knowing how to perform in clinical encounters is the first step. This is that point at which being able to evaluate your own performance (self-evaluation) accurately and realistically is vital. It is only when you are aware of your own behavior that changes to improve performance can be made. When good self-evaluation skills have been developed, it is then possible to become independent. It is hoped that this book has sparked your interest in developing good self-evaluation skills and has put you well on the course to functioning effectively as your own supervisor.

KNOW IT! USE IT!

After reading this chapter, you should be able to:

1. state at least five reasons for engaging in self-evaluation.
2. state at least five techniques you can use to help self-evaluate your performance.
3. state at least six basic clinical behaviors you will include in your initial self-evaluations.
4. state at least 30 higher level clinical behaviors you will eventually incorporate into your self-evaluations.

REFERENCES

American Speech-Language-Hearing Association. (1985). Clinical supervision in speech-language pathology and audiology. *Asha, 27,* 57–60.

Anderson, J.L. (1988a). *The supervisory process in speech-language pathology and audiology.* Boston: College-Hill Press.

Anderson, J.L. (1988b). Foreword. In P.L. Casey, K.J. Smith, & S.R. Ulrich (Eds.), *Self-supervision: A career tool for audiologists and speech-language pathologists* (pp. vii–viii). Rockville, MD: National Student Speech Language Hearing Association.

Bernthal, J.E., & Beukelman, D.R. (1975). Self-evaluation by the student clinician. *Journal of the National Student Speech and Hearing Association, 3,* 39–44.

Brasseur, J., & Jimenez, B. (1994). Supervisee self-analysis and changes in clinical behavior. In M. Bruce (Ed.), *Proceedings of the 1994 International & Interdisciplinary Conference on Clinical Supervision: Toward the 21st Century* (pp. 111–125). Houston, TX: University of Houston.

Casey, P.L., Smith, K.J., & Ulrich, S.R. (1988). *Self-supervision: A career tool for audiologists and speech-language pathologists.* Rockville, MD: National Student Speech Language Hearing Association.

Dowling, S. (1992). *Implementing the supervisory process.* Englewood Cliffs, NJ: Prentice-Hall.

McLeod, S. (1994). Student Self-Appraisal: Facilitating mutual planning in clinical education. *Clinical Supervisor, 15(1),* 87–101.

Mowrer, D. (1973). A behavioristic approach to modification of articulation. In W. Wolfe & D. Goulding (Eds.), *Articulation and learning.* Springfield, IL: Charles C Thomas.

Mowrer, D. (1988). *Methods of modifying speech behaviors* (2nd ed.). Prospect Heights, IL: Waveland Press, Inc.

Shriberg, L., Filley, F., Hayes, D., et al. (1975). The Wisconsin procedure for appraisal of clinical competence (W-PACC): Model and data. *Asha, 17,* 158–165.

Van Riper, C. (1965). Supervision of clinical practice. *Asha, 3,* 75–77.

The Basics Are Not Enough

This book has presented a comprehensive overview of how you, as beginning speech-language clinicians, can be successful in your clinical endeavors. This book has presented topical areas in which you must demonstrate competence. Frequent use of the book should help you make an easier, smoother, and more graceful transition from the context of learning (the classroom) to the context of application (clinical setting).

If you have read this book and if you continue to rely on it, you will have already been introduced to the most troublesome pitfalls, both large and small, that have perplexed many, if not all, former beginning clinicians. It is hoped that the suggestions to prevent falling into these traps have been helpful. When basic clinical procedures have been mastered, the journey is not over. You must proceed to a higher level of competence at which knowledge and application of more complex clinical procedures are necessary. Clearly, you must continue to obtain, apply, and evaluate new knowledge throughout your professional career.

Most university programs provide you with the basics of the profession in an ideal, but somewhat unrealistic, environment. The first clinical experience is usually performed in the university's in-house clinic. Clients are frequently seen on an individual basis. This environment is conducive to learning the basics about the clinical process and applying the information previously learned in lectures and text books. Once the basics have been mastered, one must learn to work with clients with less common and more complex problems.

Even in this somewhat friendly and structured environment, all services must be provided as competently and as professionally as possible. According to the ASHA code of ethics (1997, p. 71), "Individuals shall provide all services competently" (p. 71) and "Individuals shall engage in only those aspects of the professions that are within the scope of their competence, considering their level of education, training, and experience" (p. 72). It is your professional responsibility to be competent in a particular area of service delivery prior to providing services in that area, regardless of the clinical setting. To do this, you must be current and knowledge-able in the field.

Speech-language pathology as a profession is constantly changing. It is the re-sponsibility of each professional to keep up with these changes and to change with the times when appropriate. Similarly, it is the responsibility of each professional to upgrade his or her knowledge base continuously. This can be done by attending workshops presented by the various regional speech-language pathology associa-tions or by other sponsors such as hospitals, universities, and rehabilitation centers. This state-of-the-art knowledge can also be obtained by attending conventions held by state associations or by the American Speech-Language-Hearing Association. Regular reading of journals and books in speech-language pathology will also help you keep abreast of new developments. You have an obligation to get actively involved in the profession. If you have not yet become a member of the National Student Speech-Language-Hearing Association (NSSLHA), which is the student branch of ASHA, do so immediately. [Note: the NSSLHA address is the same as ASHA's, which is 10801 Rockville Pike, Rockville, Maryland 20852.] The ben-efits are numerous, but most important, you will receive journals at a substantially discounted price.

It is important not only to keep up with the trends but also to anticipate them. Because of a change in demographics, the need for services to the elderly is in-creasing. Cornett and Chabon (1988) state that "by the year 2000, 25% of persons over age 65 are expected to have a speech or language impairment, and 46% may have a hearing impairment" (p. 197). It is also necessary to keep abreast of the continuing evolution of technology in our profession. You need to keep pace with new developments and learn to use appropriate tools to enhance some or all phases of clinical practice.

In a related vein, it is also important to prepare for the geographic area where you will work. Learn as much as possible about the population that you will be serving. Specifically, learn about the cultural and linguistic diversity of the populations you will most likely encounter because it is not possible to evaluate or treat clients effectively without this important knowledge.

It is your professional responsibility to know and adhere to the regulations gov-erning your performance. All professionals in the field of speech-language pathol-ogy must be aware of the American Speech-Language-Hearing Association's code of ethics (1997, pp. 71–73) and scope of practice (pp. 74–77) as well as its various position papers. You must also be aware of legislation affecting our profession. If employed in an educational setting, it is necessary to keep abreast of special educa-tion regulations. You should be familiar with areas that impact on our positions such as outcome-based education, curriculum-based assessment, inclusion, instructional support teams, collaborative problem solving, collaborative consultation, whole language, classroom-based assessment, and classroom-based treatment. Regardless of your future employment setting, be it the schools, private practice, or some branch of health care (hospitals; long-term care such as inpatient institutional care, day hospitals, rehabilitation centers, adult day-care programs; community group homes; home care; community clinics; health maintenance organizations; preferred provider organizations, and so forth), it is of utmost importance to be aware of all the legislation, regulations, and insurance that impact on your position. It is important to be on the cutting edge of new developments. In all, it is important to keep an open mind and remain flexible—you must recognize, understand, and welcome change. Do not look at changing times or trends with fear but derive comfort from the fact that you are prepared to meet them!

REFERENCES

American Speech-Language-Hearing Association. (1997). *Membership & certification handbook: Speech-language pathology.* Rockville, MD: American Speech-Language-Hearing Association.

Cornett, B.S., & Chabon, S.S. (1988). *The clinical practice of speech-language pathology.* Columbus, OH: Merrill.

Glossary

Accountability (Clinical). Having complete, accurate, thorough records for the clients you are servicing. This means that all the required *Paperwork (Daily Log, Evaluation, Re-Evaluation, Progress Report,* as applicable) is thorough, accurate, and complete. Also refers to keeping track of your clinical hours to count toward your *Certificate of Clinical Competence* and for possible legal entanglements.

Articulation. The production of individual phonemes. Use of the articulators (lips, tongue, teeth, and so forth) to produce speech sounds.

Artificial Reinforcement. Reinforcement that does not naturally occur in the environment. Artificial reinforcers may include clapping, hugging, dispensing tokens, and so forth when a client correctly responds. This method will not teach the client the power of communication. See *Naturalistic Reinforcement, Power of Communication.*

ASHA. Acronym for the American Speech-Language-Hearing Association, the national organization for speech-language pathologists. It is located at 10801 Rockville Pike, Rockville, MD 20852-3279.

Assessment. The evaluation of a client's speech, language, and overall communicative ability. Related to *Accountability.*

Attending Behavior. The ability of a client to focus on a task.

Augmentative Device. A device or physical object used to supplement communication. It may be of high- or low-technological sophistication.

Background Information. Information you obtain about a client. Pertinent background information appears at the beginning of the written evaluation. This may include referral source, previous therapy, speech and language milestones, developmental milestones, birth history, medical history, educational history, and vocational history pending the client's age and nature of the problem.

Beginning Clinician. See *Clinician.*

Behavioral Objectives. Performance or behavior that the client is supposed to exhibit at some point in the therapy process. A behavioral objective should contain three components: performance, condition, and criterion. Behavioral objectives are found in lesson plans, evaluations, re-evaluations, and progress reports. They contribute to clinical accountability. Objectives may be revised as clients progress from one level to another. See *Long-Range Objectives, Objectives, Session Objectives, Short-Range Objectives, Short-Term Instructional Objectives, Terminal Objectives, Therapeutic Objectives,* and *Transitional Objectives.*

Branch Step. A therapy objective of lesser complexity than the one on which the client did not have success. Breaking the objective down into its component parts so that the client will have success.

CAA. Acronym for The Council on Academic Accreditation in Audiology and Speech-Language Pathology, a body of *ASHA* that defines the standards for the accreditation of graduate educational programs.

Carry Over. Using a newly learned speech, language, or communication technique in everyday situations.

CCC-A. Certificate of clinical competence in audiology.

CCC-SLP. Certificate of clinical competence in speech-language pathology.

Certificate of Clinical Competence (CCC). Granted by *ASHA* to those persons who qualify by meeting specific requirements with regard to degree, coursework, practicum, supervised professional experience and pass the national examination in speech-language pathology.

Client. A person (patient) receiving therapy from a speech-language pathologist.

Clinical Strategy Outline. A plan for a therapy session that includes *Objectives (Long-Range Objectives, Session Objectives, Short-Range Objectives)* and procedures to be used to meet those objectives. Sometimes, materials to be used are indicated. Same as a lesson plan, instructional plan, or pretherapy plan. Related to *Accountability.*

Clinician. A person providing speech and language therapy. A *beginning clinician* is one who is in a training program, is enrolled in clinical practicum, and is providing services in the area of speech, language and/or communication.

Continuous Reinforcement. Reinforcement that follows every correct response. This type of reinforcement is best for establishing a new skill or behavior.

Covert Verb. Relevant to the performance component of *Behavioral Objectives.* A verb referring to performance or behavior that cannot be directly observed. Examples include "recognize," "infer," "analyze," "recall," "identify," "solve," and "know." See *Overt Verb.*

Daily Log. A record of the client's performance during therapy sessions. Same as *progress note.* Related to *Accountability.*

Data Sheet. The paper on which the clinician records the client's responses or their outcomes. Same as *record sheet, response sheet,* and *tally sheet.* Related to *Accountability.*

Dependency (Fostering). When the clinician shares the client's problem and behaviors by encouraging the client to perform tasks for the benefit of the clinician and not for the client's betterment. The clinician often exhibits authoritarian behavior and does not encourage the client to be responsible for his problem or therapy program.

Education for All Handicapped Children Act (1975). The first compulsory special education law; mandates a free and appropriate education for all students with handicaps, between the ages of 3 and 21. Also called P.L. 94-142.

Evaluation. The written assessment of a person's speech, language, or communication abilities. Part of the *Paperwork* process and part of *Accountability.*

Expressive Language. Encoding language. The production of language. Communicating through the spoken or printed word or other forms of language.

Fixed-Ratio Reinforcement. A type of intermittent reinforcement. Reinforcement occurs after a fixed number of correct responses. It may occur after every three correct responses, or after every five correct responses, and so forth.

Fluency. The smooth, effortless, uninterrupted flow of speech.

Group Therapy. A type of therapy in which all clients in the group are interacting. Sometimes, this interaction involves non–goal-related activities or goal-related activities. This latter type is the more desirable form, although it takes more planning to achieve. See *Therapy in a Group.*

Hours Sheet. The paper on which the clinician records the amount of time spent in therapy working with various types of disorders. Same as *tracking sheet.* Related to *Accountability.*

Indicator Behavior. This is used to clarify the performance portion of a behavioral objective when a *Covert Verb* is used. The indicator behavior appears in parentheses. For example "identify (point to) pictures receptively."

Individualized Education Program (IEP). A written document required by the **Education for All Handicapped Children Act** of 1975 for every child with a disability. It must include present performance, annual goals, short-term instructional objectives, specific educational services needed, relevant dates, regular education program participation, and evaluation procedures. Is a part of *Accountability*.

Informant. The person providing background information on the client. Pending the situation, it is possible for the client to be his or her own informant.

Initial Evaluation. The first time a person's speech, language or communication abilities are assessed or the first time the clinician is evaluating the person. Part of *Accountability*.

Instructional Plan. See *Clinical Strategy Outline*.

Intermittent Reinforcement. A type of reinforcement schedule that produces greater resistance to extinction. This type of reinforcement is best for maintaining a behavior. See *Continuous Reinforcement*.

Language. The relationship between sound and meaning. A socially shared code that represents ideas through arbitrary symbols and rules that govern combinations of these symbols. A systematic set of symbols used in various modes for communication and thought.

Language Assessment. Using both formal and informal procedures to determine at what level the person is functioning with regard to the mastery of language. Both *Receptive Language* and *Expressive Language* are evaluated and included in the *Initial Evaluation* and *Re-Evaluation*. Related to *Accountability*.

Lesson Objectives. See *Session Objectives*.

Lesson Plan. See *Clinical Strategy Outline*.

Long-Range Objectives. The outcome that the clinician is guiding the client to achieve at a distant point in time. The time frame varies pending the setting. In a university setting, the time frame is defined as a semester. See also *Behavioral Objectives, Lesson Objectives, Session Objectives, Short-Range Objectives, Short-Term Instructional Objectives, Short-Term Objectives, Subobjectives, Terminal Objectives, Therapeutic Objectives,* and *Transitional Objectives*.

Long-Term Objectives. See *Long-Range Objectives*.

Monitor. Determining the correctness or incorrectness of a behavior.

Naturalistic Reinforcement. A powerful type of reinforcement. Naturally occurs in the environment. Includes getting and keeping an adult's attention, getting wants and needs met, and so on. See *Artificial Reinforcement, Power of Communication*.

NSSLHA. Acronym for the National Student Speech-Language-Hearing Association, the national organization for students majoring in speech-language pathology and audiology. It is located at 10801 Rockville Pike, Rockville, MD 20852-3279.

Objectives. Goals set for client performance. Usually in a specific order but may be altered to suit client progress. See also *Behavioral Objectives, Lesson Objectives, Long-Range Objectives, Long-Term Objectives, Session Objectives, Short-Range Objectives, Short-Term Instructional Objectives, Short-Term Objectives, Subobjectives, Terminal Objectives, Therapeutic Objectives,* and *Transitional Objectives*.

Overt Verb. Relevant to the performance component of a behavioral objective. This refers to performance that is directly observable through vision or audition. Examples are "list," "name," "point," "write," and "repeat," and so forth. See *Covert Verb*.

Paperwork. That which you must do, cannot avoid, and will never outlive. It is a relative term because the type of documents referred to vary among service providers. Within university programs, it usually refers to some or all of the following: writing *Behavioral Objectives, Evaluations, Re-evaluations, Lesson Plans, Progress Notes, Clinical Strategy Outline, Daily Log, Semester Plan of Treatment, Session Evaluation,* and *Progress Report*. The bedrock of clinical accountability that can have professional or legal implications. See *Accountability*.

Phonology. The study of the sound system of the language. It includes speech sounds (phonemes), speech patterns, and the rules that apply to these sounds.

P.L. 94-142. See *Education for All Handicapped Children Act*.

Power of Communication. Learning that the environment can be manipulated through talking. Usage of naturalistic reinforcement helps to convey this idea. See *Naturalistic Reinforcement*.

Pragmatics. The use of language in social context.

Pretherapy Plan. See *Clinical Strategy Outline*.

Problem Behavior. Behavior that interferes with the client's achievement of the objectives. For example, inattentiveness, not following directions, refusing to perform tasks, kicking, shouting, biting, and so forth.

Progress Note. See *Daily Log*.

Progress Report. A report written after the client has received therapy for a period of time. The actual amount of time that lapses varies pending the setting. In a university setting, this report is usually written at the end of the semester. The purpose is to document any improvement that has been made. Related to *Accountability*.

Receptive Language. Decoding language. Understanding or comprehending spoken or written messages as well as other forms of language.

Record Sheet. See *Data Sheet*.

Re-Evaluation. To evaluate the client again to obtain additional information, to determine whether the previous diagnosis has changed or remains accurate, or to obtain additional information about how to proceed with the client's therapy program. A type of report. Related to *Accountability*.

Reinforcement. The procedure of following a correct response with a reinforcer. See *Continuous Reinforcement, Intermittent Reinforcement*.

Response Sheet. See *Data Sheet*.

Self-Evaluation. The ability to analyze critically your professional performance accurately and in depth in order to improve your clinical skills and be the best clinician you can.

Self-Monitoring. When the client independently evaluates the correctness and incorrectness of his responses. This is a step toward the client's becoming independent. This procedure assists with the carryover process. See *Carry Over, Dependency*.

Semantics. The study of the meaning of language. This includes meaning at the word, sentence, and conversational level.

Semester (or Quarter) Plan of Treatment. This plan is specific to the university setting owing to the reference to "semester" or "quarter" and is composed of both long-range goals and short-term objectives. It is based on both formal and informal testing as well as observations formulated during the initial evaluation. Related to *Accountability.*

Session. When the clinician and client are involved in therapy.

Session Evaluation. A critique of the session upon completion. Some things to include are whether or not the objectives were met, if the procedures were helpful or not, if progress was made, what could have been done differently, strengths of the session, weaknesses of the session, and changes to be made for the next session. It may be required that this session evaluation be written on the back of the lesson plan. Sometimes it also needs to be presented verbally while conferencing with your supervisor. Related to *Accountability.*

Session Objectives. Objectives to be addressed in a specific session. Also called *lesson objectives.* See also *Short-Range Objectives.*

Short-Range Objectives. Those objectives that are attainable in a short period of time. In some settings, this period may be one session, one week, or one month. Also called *short-term objectives.* See also *Behavioral Objectives, Lesson Objectives, Long-Term Objectives, Clinical Strategy Outline, Long-Range Objectives, Session Objectives, Short-Term Instructional Objectives, Short-Term Objectives, Subobjectives, Terminal Objectives, Therapeutic Objectives,* and *Transitional Objectives.*

Short-Term Instructional Objectives. Required by law for *Individualized Education Program.* See also *Session Objectives.*

Short-Term Objectives. See *Short-Range Objectives.*

Smothering (the Client). Using language that is beyond the client's expressive language ability.

Speech-Language Pathologist. A person holding a degree and certification in speech-language pathology who is qualified to diagnose and treat speech, language, voice, and communication problems. Holds state licensure.

Speech-Language Pathology Assistant. Support personnel in speech-language pathology who can perform tasks as prescribed, directed, and supervised by certified speech-language pathologists following academic and/or on-the-job training. Credentialing for assistants is done through *ASHA* but differs from that for speech-language pathologists.

Student Self-Appraisal. A procedure that helps students self-evaluate and reflect on their clinical experiences.

Subobjectives. See *Session Objectives.*

Subjective, Objective, Assessment, and Plan (SOAP). One format for writing progress notes.

Tally Sheet. See *Data Sheet.*

Terminal Objectives. Those objectives that need to be accomplished prior to the client's discharge from therapy. See *Behavioral Objectives, Lesson Objectives, Long-Range Objectives, Session Objectives, Short-Range Objectives, Short-Term Instructional Objectives, Short-Term Objectives, Subobjectives, Therapeutic Objectives,* and *Transitional Objectives.*

Therapy. The process whereby the clinician guides the client in working on and meeting his objectives. The process of guiding the client from his current level of functioning to the level at which he should be functioning.

Therapy in a Group. When the clinician provides individual therapy to each of the clients in a group setting. See *Group Therapy.*

Therapy Program. The plan through which the speech-language pathologist guides the client in order to remediate or decrease the severity of his or her problem. Related to *Accountability.*

Therapeutic Objectives. The objectives that should be focused on in therapy. See *Behavioral Objectives, Lesson Objectives, Long-Range Objectives, Long-Term Objectives, Objectives, Session Objectives, Short-Range Objectives, Short-Term Instructional Objectives, Short-Term Objectives, Subobjectives, Terminal Objectives,* and *Transitional Objectives.*

Tracking Sheet. See *Hours Sheet.*

Transitional Objectives. Session objectives presented in a specific order, subject to alteration based on client performance. See *Session Objectives.*

Treatment Plan. A plan for a therapy session that includes objectives *(Short-Term Objectives)* and procedures to be used to meet these objectives. Sometimes, materials are included. Same as a *clinical strategy outline, instructional plan,* or *lesson plan.* Related to *Accountability.*

Voice. Sound produced by the vibration of the vocal folds and modified by the resonators (oral cavity, nasal cavity, pharynx, and so on).

Index

V

W